Innovative Approaches for Safety Culture Improvement in Healthcare Systems

Innovative Approaches for Safety Culture Improvement in Healthcare Systems

Guest Editors

Marie E. Ward
Eva Doherty
Siobhán Corrigan

MDPI

Basel • Beijing • Wuhan • Barcelona • Belgrade • Novi Sad • Cluj • Manchester

Guest Editors

Marie E. Ward
Health Systems Learning and Research
St James's Hospital
Dublin
Ireland

Eva Doherty
Department of Surgical Affairs
RCSI University of Medicine and Health Sciences
Dublin
Ireland

Siobhán Corrigan
Centre for Innovative Human Systems (CIHS)
Trinity College Dublin
Dublin
Ireland

Editorial Office
MDPI AG
Grosspeteranlage 5
4052 Basel, Switzerland

This is a reprint of the Special Issue, published open access by the journal *Healthcare* (ISSN 2227-9032), freely accessible at: https://www.mdpi.com/journal/healthcare/special_issues/C5M46LAD0V.

For citation purposes, cite each article independently as indicated on the article page online and as indicated below:

Lastname, A.A.; Lastname, B.B. Article Title. *Journal Name* **Year**, *Volume Number*, Page Range.

ISBN 978-3-7258-5053-2 (Hbk)
ISBN 978-3-7258-5054-9 (PDF)
https://doi.org/10.3390/books978-3-7258-5054-9

Cover image courtesy of Marie E. Ward

Contents

About the Editors

Marie E. Ward

Marie E. Ward, BA (Hons), PhD, C.ErgHF, FCIEHF, MIHFES, is an embedded researcher at St James's Hospital, Dublin, Ireland, where she is engaged in a programme of Health Systems and Human Factors Ergonomics Research and Improvement. Marie holds a PhD in Psychology Human Factors from Trinity College Dublin (TCD) and is an Adjunct Assistant Professor at TCD's multidisciplinary Centre for Innovative Human Systems, which engages in Human Factors research and consultancy with all industries to improve human wellbeing and system performance. Marie is a lecturer on the Masters in Managing Risk and System Change (TCD) and the Masters in Human Factors in Patient Safety courses at the Royal College of Surgeons Ireland (RCSI); the Chairperson of the Irish Human Factors and Ergonomics Society; a member of the Chartered Institute of Ergonomics and Human Factors (UK) special interest group on Artificial Intelligence in Healthcare; and a Chartered Ergonomist and Human Factors Specialist. Her research interests include co-designing new systems from a socio-technical perspective to enable patient and staff safety and wellbeing, and system performance. Marie has co-authored over 120 peer-reviewed publications and received the International Ergonomics Association Liberty Mutual Medal for outstanding original research in Human Factors Ergonomics.

Eva Doherty

Eva Doherty, DClinPsych, CClinPsychol (AFPsSI), CPsychol (AFBPsS), PFHEA, FEACH is a practising Chartered Clinical Psychologist, Associate Professor and Director of the Human Factors in Patient Safety (HFPS) training, research and assessment programmes at the National Surgical Training Centre, Department of Surgical Affairs, RCSI University of Medicine and Health Sciences, Dublin, Ireland. The HFPS training is a mandatory component of the postgraduate professional training for surgical, emergency medicine, radiology, and ophthalmology trainees. Each year, over 100 interactive workshops and high-fidelity simulation training courses are delivered to trainee doctors, doctors not currently in training, and consultants on topics which include medical error, risk management, communication, teamwork, conflict resolution, decision-making, open disclosure, emotional intelligence, crisis management, stress and wellbeing, professionalism, and leadership. Eva pioneered and directs the academic Postgraduate Diploma/MSc in Human Factors in Patient Safety, which is an inter-professional one/two-year part-time online programme. Eva has over 50 peer-reviewed publications on topics relevant to clinical communication issues, curriculum development, and personality factors in medical education and assessment. Eva acts as advisor to the National Healthcare Communication Programme in Ireland, HSE. She is a member of the ISQua Expert Panel and the Independent National Patient Safety Council in the Department of Health. In recognition of Eva's contribution to medical education and to communication training in healthcare, Eva was awarded a Principal Fellowship by the Higher Education Academy in the U.K. and an honorary fellowship by EACH International, the International Association for Communication in Healthcare.

Siobhán Corrigan

Siobhán Corrigan, BSc, MSc, PhD, is an Associate Professor in Organisational Psychology at the School of Psychology, Trinity College Dublin. She is Co-Director of the Research Centre for Innovative Human Systems (CIHS) and Director of the Postgraduate programmes in Managing Risk and System

Change (Certificate, Diploma, MSc). Her research adopts socio-technical systems approaches to enhance human and organisational performance in complex safety-critical environments, focusing specifically on managing the challenges of implementing change. Siobhán lectures in Organisational Behaviour; Change Management; Leadership, Human Factors, and Qualitative Research Methods. She has published extensively in her field and was awarded the 2024 Excellence in Research Student Supervision award for her contribution to fostering a culture of excellence in postgraduate research at Trinity College.

Preface

Improvements in patient safety have been achieved over the last twenty years, yet challenges remain in relation to safety culture, including the belief among healthcare professionals that blame is still part of their culture.

This Special Issue presents papers that explore innovative approaches to understanding and developing safety culture in healthcare. The papers included within demonstrate the importance of taking a systems perspective when considering safety culture, including understanding culture as both an emergent property of systems and something that shapes systems, and as something that can improve patient and staff safety.

Three case studies are presented in this Special Issue in relation to understanding and improving the safety culture in an intensive care unit, a nursing home, and in an obstetrics and gynecology department. Four papers present different ways to facilitate safety culture, including the importance of the patient's voice in understanding safety; the need for psychological safety among healthcare professionals to speak up for safety and a joint problem-solving orientation towards addressing problems when they are raised; the role of informal communication between healthcare professionals in joint sensemaking for safety and breaking the silence around safety; and the importance of informed consent for patients.

Two perspectives in relation to just culture are presented, including one on the unique challenges of operationalizing just culture in residential care settings and a second on enabling organizational conditions for restorative just culture.

The Guest Editors would like to take this opportunity to thank each of the contributing authors who have made this Special Issue such an interesting collection of papers on the important topic of safety culture in healthcare. We would also like to thank the peer reviewers and the Healthcare Editorial team for all their help and support.

Marie E. Ward, Eva Doherty, and Siobhán Corrigan
Guest Editors

healthcare

MDPI

Article

Exploring Safety Culture in the ICU of a Large Acute Teaching Hospital through Triangulating Different Data Sources

Ellen Liston [1,2,*], Enda O'Connor [1,3] and Marie E. Ward [1,4]

1 St James's Hospital, D08 NHY1 Dublin, Ireland; oconnoen@tcd.ie (E.O.); maward@stjames.ie (M.E.W.)
2 Department of Surgical Affairs, Royal College of Surgeons, D02 YN77 Dublin, Ireland
3 School of Medicine, Faculty of Health Sciences, Trinity College, The University of Dublin, D02 PN40 Dublin, Ireland
4 Centre for Innovative Human Systems, Trinity College, The University of Dublin, D02 PN40 Dublin, Ireland
* Correspondence: ellen.liston@hse.ie

Abstract: Safety Culture (SC) has become a key priority for safety improvement in healthcare. Studies have identified links between positive SC and improved patient outcomes. Mixed-method measurements of SC are needed to account for diverse social, cultural, and subcultural contexts within different healthcare settings. The aim of the study was to triangulate data on SC from three sources in an Intensive Care Unit (ICU) in a large acute teaching hospital. A mixed-methods approach was used, including analysing the Hospital Survey for Patient Safety Culture results, retrospective chart reviews using the Global Trigger Tool (GTT) for the ICU, and staff reporting of adverse events (AE). There was a 47% (101/216) response rate for the survey. Further, 98% of respondents stated a positive patient safety rating. The GTT identified 16 AEs and 11 AEs that were reported in the same timeframe. The triangulation of the data demonstrates the complexity of understanding components of SC in particular: learning, reporting, and just culture.

Keywords: patient safety culture; psychological safety; just culture; intensive care; acute hospital

1. Introduction

Patient Safety has been recognised as an important public health, ethical, and economic issue needing significant research and improvement initiatives since the publication of landmark reports [1]. High-profile incidents and reports in healthcare have revealed multiple systemic failures attributable to Safety Culture (SC), including poor leadership, failure to risk assess, and breakdown of teamwork [2]. SC has become a key priority for safety improvement in healthcare, despite variations in definition [3]. The WHO Global Patient Safety Action Plan emphasises the need to instil a strong safety culture into the design and delivery of healthcare to ensure a reduction in both patient and staff harm [4]. Originating in the Nuclear Power industry, the concept of SC was coined to capture a lack of individual and organisational commitment to prioritise safety [5]. Research in the largest EU-funded project on Human Factors in aviation safety, the human integration in the lifecycle of aviation systems (HILAS) programme, adapted Reason's initial five-component model of safety culture [6], to include the following seven components: (i) prioritising safety; (ii) ensuring standards and reliability; (iii) flexibility and resilience; (iv) learning culture; (v) teamwork; (vi) a reporting culture; and (vii) a just culture [7]. All these components, taken together, are important to SC [8].

Despite SC being a recognised priority, rates of patient harm have remained, if not increased, and patient safety initiatives have not systematically tackled SC within healthcare [2,9]. The diversity in healthcare organisations and systems accounts somewhat for this, but Provonost et al. argue that prioritising safety is key and taking a systems approach to do so rather than a persistent blame culture, focusing on punishment rather than learning, which appears to be characteristic of healthcare [10]. Under-reporting of incidents remains a widespread issue [11,12], and barriers to reporting identified in the literature include fear of repercussions and a lack of feedback or action when incidents are reported [13–16]. Mixed-method measurements of SC are needed to account for diverse social, cultural, and subcultural contexts within different healthcare settings [17,18] and to understand how these different components of SC play out in different settings. To date, there is no study in Ireland that has used more than one method of measurement to examine SC, specifically in the ICU.

1.1. Safety Culture in the ICU

Within hospitals, intensive care units (ICUs) are particularly high-risk areas for medical errors and adverse events (AE) that could occur due to the complexity of care and the patients' fragile medical conditions [18]. Studies have been carried out using survey and interview-based designs to explore SC in the ICU. Farzi et al. [19], for example, studied safety culture among Iranian nurses in the ICU using the Agency for Healthcare Research and Quality's (AHRQ) Hospital Survey on Patient Safety Culture (HSOPSC) and reported that nurses found "teamwork within units" and "organizational learning-continuous improvement" to be the most positive features of their safety culture. They assigned the least positive scores to "handoffs and transitions" and "non-punitive response to errors". Gomides et al. [20] evaluated perceptions of SC within an MDT of a Brazilian ICU using the Safety Attitudes Questionnaire. They found low scores for safety attitudes related to the domains of management, working conditions, and communication failures.

Tlili et al. [18] studied SC among nurses, doctors, healthcare technicians, and assistant caregivers in 15 Tunisian ICUs using the HSOPSC and follow-up interviews with 12 staff. They found all the SC dimensions had a score of less than 50%. The most widely implemented dimension was "teamwork within units". The least positive scores were assigned to "communication openness" and "non-punitive response to error".

1.2. Evaluating SC and Triangulating Data

1.2.1. SC Survey Studies

There are a limited number of studies that use more than one method to evaluate SC. Recent studies [17,21–24] have emphasised the importance of using various data collection methods to account for the complexity of SC. The most frequently used measurement tools in the SC literature are the Safety Attitudes Questionnaire and the AHRQ HSOPSC [1] surveys. Both questionnaires have been empirically tested for psychometric validity and reliability [16,25]. HSOPSC has been recommended for use in healthcare organisations to assess SC, track changes, and evaluate the impact of safety interventions [11]. The AHRQ also allows organisations to enter their results into a database that allows for the comparison of findings across similar contexts.

1.2.2. SC Mixed-Methods Studies

Mardon et al. [21] measured staff perceptions of SC and their association with AE using the HSOPSC and AHRQ Patient Safety Indicators. They found that higher SC scores tended to have fewer Patient Safety Indicators, including, for example, lower rates of in-hospital complications, and that this association remained after adjustments for hospital characteristics and measurements. More recently, Denning et al. [23] also investigated SC by studying staff perceptions of SC and staff AE reporting, specifically in response to the COVID-19 pandemic, and found there was a considerable reduction in reporting. When broken down by type, "No Harm" and "Near Miss" reports were significantly reduced during the pandemic ($p < 0.003$). However, the level of reporting for "Harm" incidents did not significantly change.

1.2.3. Adverse Event Reporting and Medical Record Review Studies

A review by Hibbert et al. [26] examined the available literature on two-stage Medical Record Reviews, as an adjunct to reported AE [26]. The two most commonly used Medical

Record Reviews in the literature are the Institute for Healthcare Improvement Global Trigger Tool (GTT) and the Harvard Method. They found that GTT is a more commonly used tool, as it is a flexible tool that can be modified to the context. Rates of AE per 100 admissions ranged from 7% to 51%, with 10% of admissions being associated with an AE [15].

The aim of this study was to explore SC in the ICU of a large acute teaching hospital through the rigorous application of three different methods and triangulating data from three sources:

(i) Staff completion of the HSOPSC survey;
(ii) Using the GTT to carry out a retrospective chart review of a sample of patient charts;
(iii) Reviewing AEs as reported by staff through the hospital electronic AE reporting system.

2. Materials and Methods

2.1. Study Setting

The study took place in the largest acute teaching hospital in Ireland, with over 1000 beds and 5000 staff. The hospital provides acute and emergency care for adult patients through a broad range of specialist medical, surgical, and oncology services. The study was completed in the 26-bed ICU of the hospital. All 216 professionals who worked in the ICU during the time of the study were invited to participate. This included nurses (staff nurses, clinical nurse managers, clinical nurse facilitators, and advanced nurse practitioners), doctors (interns, senior house officers, registrars, and consultants), health care assistants, and health and social care professionals (HSCPs) (e.g., pharmacists, speech and language therapists, clinical nutritionists, medical social workers, occupational therapists, and physiotherapists). Based on the AHRQ guidance [26], for settings with 500 or fewer staff, a 50% response rate should be expected. Therefore, the predicted response rate was 50% (108) participants.

2.2. Study Design

A mixed-methods approach was used, building on the strengths of different approaches. Information on the SC in the ICU was explored through three sources:

(i) Staff completion of the HSOPSC survey: Survey data was collected using HSOPSC version 2.0 (Supplementary File S1) approved by the AHRQ [27]. The survey contains a total of 40 survey items, divided across 10 composite measures of SC, primarily using 5-point agreement scales ("Strongly disagree" to "Strongly agree") or frequency scales ("Never" to "Always") with a "Does not apply or Don't know" option. Composites include Communication About Error, Communication Openness, Handoffs and Information Exchange, Hospital Management Support for Patient Safety, Organizational Learning-Continuous Improvement, Reporting Patient Safety Events, Response to Error, Staffing and Work Pace, Supervisor, Manager, or Clinical Leader Support for Patient Safety and Teamwork. There is also an item on patient safety events the respondent has reported and a further item seeking an overall rating on patient safety for their work unit/area. An additional open-ended question probes perceptions around overall patient safety in the hospital. The demographic data of participants were collected using the same questionnaire, identifying profession, work area, and level of experience. The wording of job roles was adapted to correlate with the Irish setting, as advised by the AHRQ guidance document.
(ii) Using the GTT to carry out a retrospective chart review of a sample of patient charts: As many studies have previously identified low rates of incident reporting [9], a retrospective chart review was completed for a two-week period. The GTT for intensive care was used (Supplementary File S2) to gather this data [28–30].
(iii) Reviewing AEs reported by staff from the ICU through the hospital electronic incident reporting system.

2.3. Data Collection Tools, Methods, and Procedures

How data was gathered using the survey, GTT, and AE analysis is outlined here:

(i) The HSOPSC, with a participant information leaflet (PIL), was distributed both electronically by email and with paper hard copies. Email links were sent by the critical care administrator, clinical nurse facilitator, and critical care lead to all staff working within the ICU at the time of the study. As the survey was completed anonymously, the Ethics Committee agreed that informed consent was implied through the completion of the survey. An additional follow-up email was sent one month later. To protect against unauthorised access, the survey link was distributed using the hospital internal email system. Hardcopies of the survey and PIL were distributed in person to all professionals working within the ICU at ward rounds, MDT meetings, and quality and audit meetings during February and March 2022.

(ii) Prior to administration of the HSOPSC samples of patients' electronic patient records (EPR) were reviewed using the GTT for predicting potential patient harm, as outlined in the Institute for Healthcare Improvement protocol [29,30]. Ten records were selected at random from all patients admitted and discharged from ICU, over a two-week period in February 2022. Patients who were admitted <24 h to ICU, under 18, and those patients with a primary psychiatric diagnosis were excluded as outlined in the Institute for Healthcare Improvement guideline. A random number generator was used to ensure random selection. Selected patient charts were anonymised on a password-protected Excel file, stored in the Principal Investigator's secure folder on the hospital's internal IT system. EPR records were reviewed for triggers initially by two reviewers, including the main author (EL) and an HSCP colleague who was familiar with the tool. Both reviewers had completed training in the use of the tool. Data was recorded on separate paper forms by each reviewer, as outlined in the Institute for Healthcare Improvement guide [30].

(iii) Reviewing AEs was carried out through an analysis of AEs reported, through the hospital electronic incident reporting system, by staff who work in the ICU. All incidents reported in February 2022 were included. Data provided to the researchers was anonymised.

The Checklist for Reporting Of Survey Studies (CROSS) quality appraisal tool for carrying out web-based and non-web-based surveys was used and can be found in the supplemental material to this article [31].

2.4. Data Analysis

How the data gathered from the three different sources was analysed is outlined here:

(i) Electronic and hard copy HSOPSC survey data were inputted into a Microsoft Excel spreadsheet created and supplied by the AHRQ. All included data were cross-checked for any errors in data entry before analysis. Responses were calculated referencing the AHRQ Guidance document [27]. Missing data and "Does not apply/Don't know" responses were excluded from calculations. Descriptive statistics were used to calculate the mean score and the average percentage of positive responses. The average percentage of positive and negative responses was calculated. The scores were reversed for negatively worded items—these are noted with an (R) after them in the survey. A One-way ANOVA was used for comparison with the AHRQ international database, with statistical significance set at $p < 0.05$. Tukey post-hoc tests were used when significance was detected. Demographic data were analysed using descriptive statistics, referencing characteristics of respondents, specifically professional experience. Qualitative data from the open-ended questions of the questionnaire were analysed using content analysis [32]. The data was systematically reviewed and highlighted where SC domains or components were referenced. This was then coded and categorised by SC domain relevance. Further examination of the data was then completed to include barriers and facilitators to patient safety and SC, coded again by SC domains. Categorisation was then completed by grouping the data by positive or negative responses. Following this systematic analysis of the data, themes were formed.

(ii) For the GTT, the triggers were examined for AE occurrence and classified in terms of harm. The National Coordination Council for Medication Error Reporting and Prevention (NCC MERP) harm categories are commonly used with the GTT [26] and include Category E: Temporary harm to the patient and required intervention; Category F: Temporary harm to the patient and required initial or prolonged Hospitalisation; Category G: Permanent patient harm Category H: Intervention required to sustain life; Category I: Patient death. After the initial review was completed separately by the two reviewers, the data were collated, and agreement was reached through consensus on rating. An ICU Consultant (EOC) then reviewed the collated data to ensure agreement on the occurrence of an AE and categorisation.

(iii) The reported AE data from the hospital electronic incident reporting systems were reviewed and incidents reported were categorised by one author (EL) according to type, level of harm, and whether the reported AE was related to patients or staff. There was no other formal method of AE reporting in the hospital at the time of the study.

3. Results

The results will initially be presented separately and then triangulated to explore the SC in the ICU from the perspective that the different data sources give us.

3.1. Hospital Survey on Patient Safety Culture Results (HSOPSC) Results

3.1.1. Demographics

A total of 101/216 questionnaires were completed from February 2022 to the end of March 2022. This equated to a 47% response rate. Table 1 shows a further breakdown of respondents by staff position. Further, 97% of respondents worked only in Intensive Care, with 2% in anaesthesiology and 1% across many different units. Staff experience varied, with 17 respondents working in the hospital less than a year, 41 respondents 1–5 years, 19 respondents 6–10 years, and 24 respondents 11 years or more. 79 respondents worked 30 to 40 h per week, with 21 working more than this. A total of 96 respondents (95%) reported having direct contact with patients.

Table 1. Breakdown of respondents by staff position.

Staff Positions	Percentage
Advanced Practice Nurse (ANP, CNS, CF, CNM)	17%
Staff Nurse	56%
Intern/SHO Doctor	4%
Registrar or Consultant Doctor	10%
Health and Social Care Professional (HSCP)	11%
Other (incl. 1 non-disclosed)	3%

Advanced Nurse Practitioner(ANP), Clinical Nurse Specialist (CNS), Clinical Facilitator (CF), Clinical Nurse Manager (CNM).

3.1.2. Survey Composites

Table 2 shows the percentages of positive, neutral, and negative responses from staff for SC composite survey items. Where the question was positively worded, answers of "Strongly Agree/Agree" and "Always/Most of the time" account for positive responses. In negatively worded questions that were reverse scored (R), answers of "Strongly Disagree/Disagree" and "Never/Rarely" account for positive responses. Negative answers were the opposite of this. Neutral responses account for answers of "Neither Agree nor Disagree/Sometimes". Where a respondent answered "Does not know" or "Does not Apply" their answer was not included in the percentage.

Table 2. Breakdown of HSOPSC responses per survey question.

	Positive %	Neutral %	Negative %
Supervisor, Manager or Clinical Leader Support for Patient Safety			
1. My supervisor, manager, or clinical leader seriously considers staff suggestions for improving patient safety.	84	12	4
2. My supervisor, manager, or clinical leader wants us to work faster during busy times, even if it means taking shortcuts. (R)	77	15	8
3. My supervisor, manager, or clinical leader takes action to address patient safety concerns that are brought to their attention.	93	6	1
Teamwork			
1. In this unit, we work together as an effective team.	97	2	1
2. During busy times, staff in this unit help each other.	97	3	0
3. There is a problem with disrespectful behaviour by those working in this unit. (R)	76	12	12
Communication Openness			
1. In this unit, staff speak up if they see something that may negatively affect patient care.	76	21	3
2. When staff in this unit see someone with more authority doing something unsafe for patients, they speak up.	49	29	22
3. When staff in this unit speak up, those with more authority are open to their patient safety concerns.	66	30	4
4. In this unit, staff are afraid to ask questions when something does not seem right. (R)	55	38	7
Reporting Patient Safety Events			
1. When a mistake is caught and corrected before reaching the patient, how often is this reported?	45	28	28
2. When a mistake reaches the patient and could have harmed the patient but did not, how often is this reported?	71	18	10
Organizational Learning—Continuous Improvement			
1. This unit regularly reviews work processes to determine if changes are needed to improve patient safety.	78	14	8
2. In this unit, changes to improve patient safety are evaluated to see how well they worked.	75	16	9
3. This unit lets the same patient safety problems keep happening (R)	80	9	12
Communication About Error			
1. We are informed about errors that happen in this unit.	51	39	10
2. When errors happen in this unit, we discuss ways to prevent them from happening again.	68	25	7
3. In this unit, we are informed about changes that are made based on event reports.	56	31	13
Hospital Management Support for Patient Safety			
1. The actions of hospital management show that patient safety is a top priority.	66	22	12
2. Hospital management provides adequate resources to improve patient safety.	63	15	23
3. Hospital management seems interested in patient safety only after an adverse event happens. (R)	25	17	58

Table 2. *Cont.*

	Positive %	Neutral %	Negative %
Response To Error			
1. In this unit, staff feel like their mistakes are held against them. (R)	61	22	18
2. When an event is reported in this unit, it feels like the person is being written up, not the problem. (R)	62	14	24
3. When staff make errors, this unit focuses on learning rather than blaming individuals.	66	20	14
4. In this unit, there is a lack of support for staff involved in patient safety errors. (R)	67	21	12
Handoffs and Information Exchange			
1. When transferring patients from one unit to another, important information is often left out. (R)	47	16	37
2. During shift changes, important patient care information is often left out. (R)	74	12	15
3. During shift changes, there is adequate time to exchange all key patient care information.	77	7	16
Staffing and Work Pace			
1. In this unit, we have enough staff to handle the workload.	50	11	40
2. Staff in this unit work longer hours than is best for patient care. (R)	32	23	44
3. This unit relies too much on temporary, float, or PRN staff. (R)	60	25	15
4. The work pace in this unit is so rushed that it negatively affects patient safety. (R)	62	19	19

	Positively worded	Negatively Worded (R)
Positive	"Strongly Agree/Agree" "Always/Most of the time"	"Strongly Disagree/Disagree" "Never/Rarely"
Neutral	"Neither Agree nor Disagree/Sometimes".	"Neither Agree nor Disagree/Sometimes".
Negative	"Strongly Disagree/Disagree" "Never/Rarely"	"Strongly Agree/Agree" "Always/Most of the time"

Figure 1 shows the average positive response of respondents for each of the 10 SC composites contained in the survey, in comparison to the AHRQ database (172 entries in the database as of December 2021). The Kolmogorov-Smirnov statistical test was performed on both data sets and found the data to be normally distributed. One-way ANOVA tests were completed using IBM® SPSS® Version 26. Results showed differences were not statistically significant (p = 0.07–0.277), and post-hoc Tukey tests were therefore not performed.

In the Teamwork composite, there was an overall 90% positive response, with the included individual question responses in the MAX category. Composites of communication openness, reporting patient safety events, communication about errors, and hospital management support for patient safety were at least 10% below the average. When compared to data for the ICU, this only applied to the composites of communication openness and reporting patient safety events.

Individual questions in Communication openness scored 6% below the minimal recorded on the database and 23% below the average for "When staff in this unit see someone with more authority doing something unsafe for patients, they speak up". For "In this unit, staff are afraid to ask questions when something doesn't seem right" the responses were 16% below average. These relate to the SC component of just culture. In "Reporting Patient Safety Events" the individual question "When a mistake is caught and corrected before reaching the patient, how often is this reported" scored 20% below the average (45%)—this is related to the SC component of reporting culture and in particular reporting of "near misses".

Communication about Error scored 19% below the average for "We are informed about errors that happen in this unit". In "Hospital Management Support for Patient Safety", the individual statement "Hospital management seems interested in patient safety only after an adverse event happens" scored 24% below the average positive response, with a 58% negative response.

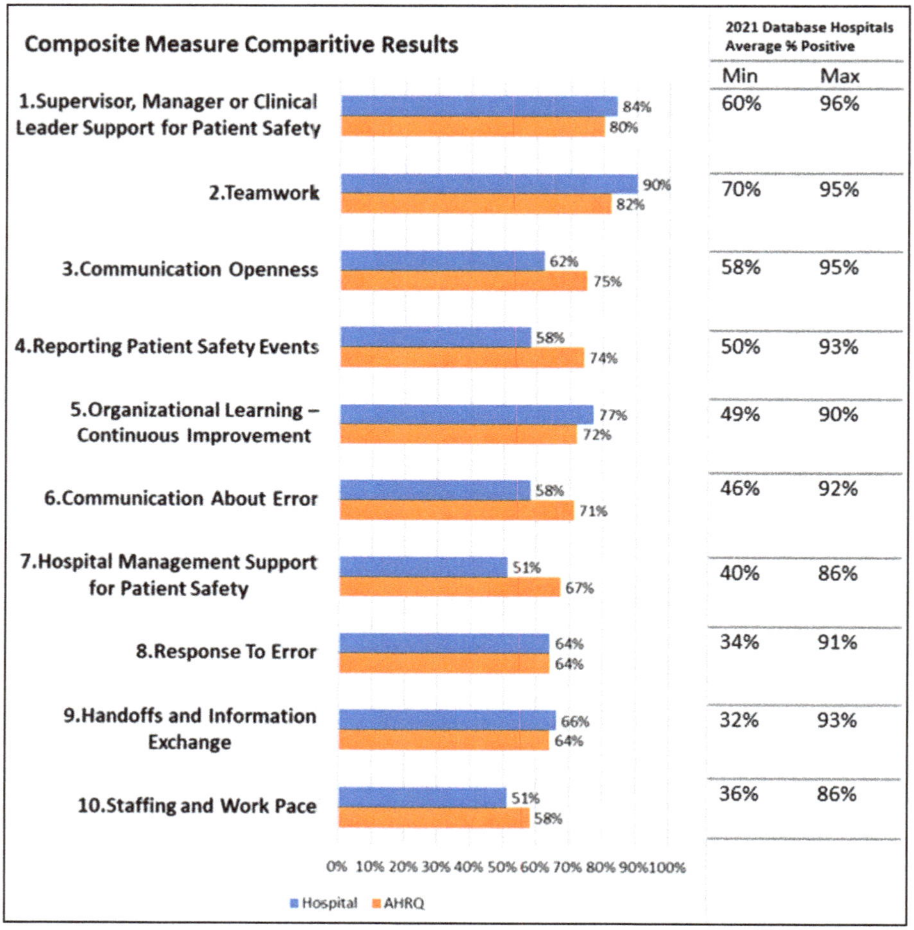

Figure 1. AHRQ database vs. study results composite comparison.

3.1.3. Safety Rating

A total of 98% of respondents reported at least a good safety rating, of whom 48% reported a very good rating, 15% excellent, and 35% good. These were compared favourably to AHRQ data (91% of respondents reported positively, 7% reported fair, and 2% reported poor). When adjusted to ICU specifically, there was a slight increase to 10% of fair responses and 3% of poor responses; however, again, the most common rating was very good (41%).

3.1.4. Number of Events Reported

Here, 48% of respondents had not completed an incident report in the preceding 12 months, 37% had completed 1–2 reports, and 14% had completed more than two. This was comparable to the AHRQ database, with a slight increase in those reporting more than two when adjusted to the ICU specifically (26%).

3.1.5. Qualitative Data

Here, 18% (n = 18) of respondents completed the open-ended question (Table 3). Content analysis was carried out on the responses, identifying both positive and negative themes and categorising them based on the safety culture domains where relevant.

Of the responses to the open-ended qualitative question, there was one positive comment relating to teamwork; the other 17 comments were either negative or suggestions for change. The themes for these related to staffing concerns (n = 7), communication (n = 5), reporting culture (n = 3), equipment (n = 2), and others (2).

Table 3. Sample qualitative comments.

Sample Qualitative Comments		**Staff Category**
Teamwork positive comment	"Fantastic teamwork between all forms of staff."	Other/Not disclosed
Staffing Concerns	"Adequate staffing would positively impact patient safety, ensuring they are receiving the correct level of care".	Health & Social Care Professional (HSCP)
Communication	"I would also like to see a clear follow through and delivery of information to staff. How many near misses/adverse events etc. and what is being done to minimise further incidents"	Advanced Nurse Practitioner (ANP, CNS, CF, CNM) *
Reporting Culture	"I have been blamed for putting too many incident reports, so now avoid them as far as possible."	Staff Nurse
Equipment	"Sometimes lack of equipment, bed spaces too small/not fit for purpose can cause safety concerns, which are well known, but little has changed."	Staff Nurse

* Advanced Nurse Practitioner(ANP), Clinical Nurse Specialist (CNS), Clinical Facilitator (CF), Clinical Nurse Manager (CNM).

3.2. AE Results

In total, there were 11 reported AEs related to the ICU for February 2022 (Table 4). Of these, six related to pressure ulcers, two to medication safety, two to device/equipment faults, and one to a reported occupational health injury. Further, 10 (90%) of these events affected patients, with the remaining incident affecting a staff member. The AEs ranged in severity from near miss (n = 1) to harm events (n = 10). The reported pressure ulcers were of low grade and acquired during the patient's ICU stay.

Table 4. Breakdown of AEs.

	AE Data	**GTT**
ICU admissions	123	123
Charts reviewed	-	10
Triggers	-	43
No. of events	11	16
Near miss	1	0
Temp harm	3	15
Harm	7	1
Medication-related	2	6

In the hospital, medication-related harm is separated from other types of harm and categorised using the NCC MERP index for categorising medication errors. Of the two medication-safety AEs, one was classified as a MERP category "C" (An error occurred that reached the patient but did not cause patient harm) and one as a MERP category "E" (An error occurred that may have contributed to or resulted in temporary harm to the patient and required intervention).

3.3. GTT Results

Of the 10 charts reviewed using the GTT, a total of 43 triggers were identified, with a median number of 4 per chart (range 2–7). From this, 16 AEs were identified (Table 4); the median was 2 per chart (range 0–4), and 2 charts (20%) contained no adverse events. 15 of the 16 AEs were rated as NCC MERP category E (temporary harm to the patient and required intervention) and 1 category F (temporary harm to the patient and required readmission to the ICU or prolonged hospitalisation either in the ICU or step-down units). Six of the AEs were related to medication, including antibiotics, anticoagulants/antiplatelets, insulin, and narcotics. The severity of harm from these events was: 1 MERP category "C" (An error occurred that reached the patient but did not cause patient harm); 3 MERP category "D" (An error occurred that reached the patient and required monitoring to confirm that it resulted in no harm to the patient and/or required intervention to preclude harm); 2 MERP category "E" (An error occurred that may have contributed to or resulted in temporary harm to the patient and required intervention). The median length of stay in the ICU in the charts included was 6.5 days (range 1–14).

3.4. Triangulation of Data

3.4.1. HSOPSC and AE Data

The triangulation of data relates most to the SC components of learning, reporting, and just culture. When the composites from HSOPSC were explored in more detail, it could be seen that 'reporting patient safety events' is at 58%, 16% below the average AHRQ score. Participants were also asked about their own AE reporting behaviour in the survey. 48% of respondents reported that they had not completed an incident report in the last 12 months, with 37% of respondents stating they had completed 1–2 and 14% of respondents stating they had completed more than two. Taken together this roughly works out for staff noting that they report about one AE every 4 days. The actual AE reported data for a two-week timeframe was 11 AEs reported—this corresponds to nearly one AE every day. So staff reported more AEs to the hospital AE reporting system than they noted in the HSOPSC that they do. However, reporting may be below the national average. Reported AEs at the same time point showed a 9% occurrence, 3% lower in comparison to large-scale published Irish studies [14]. While not directly comparable, due to the small data set, it may demonstrate an underreporting of AEs within the study setting.

3.4.2. GTT and AE Data

When we compare the GTT results with the reported AEs, we find that 16 AEs were identified in the GTT, none of which were reported as AEs through the hospital incident reporting system. None of the reported AEs (11) through the hospital system were the same events as the AEs identified using the GTT (16). This might help explain the perception of staff that they underreport AEs. Staff may realise that more AEs are taking place than they report, and this may be related to the nature of the AEs (e.g., near misses). In February 2022, there were 123 admissions to the General Intensive Care Unit. The GTT data therefore represents 8% of these admissions. Within the 8% represented, an AE occurred in 80% (n = 8) of charts reviewed using the GTT. Further, 94% of the AEs identified through the GTT caused temporary or no harm to the patient, which may account for some of these events not being reported. For example, specifically focusing on medication-related events, there were two events reported in February 2022, whereas the GTT data identified six medication safety events within the data set, none of which were the same as the reported events. As stated above, four of these events did not cause harm to the patient, with the other two causing temporary harm, which may account for them not being reported.

4. Discussion

The survey data demonstrate an overall positive SC, with 5 out of the 10 composites scoring the same as, above, or well above the international benchmark. Areas of Teamwork, Supervisor/Manager/Clinical leader support for patient safety; Organisational learning/Continuous improvement; and Handoffs information exchange scored above 75% positive responses, at the upper range when benchmarked against the AHRQ database. In the 2022 report of OECD countries, including over 20 countries, 68% of health workers reported high levels of teamwork, and 65% stated their organisation exhibited positive continuous improvement [1]. For the study population, there was a 22% higher positive response for Teamwork and 12% for Continuous Improvement. This demonstrates a willingness to support and work effectively together towards improved patient outcomes, evaluate and implement change, and take action to prevent AEs [27]. The SC dimensions of teamwork, ensuring standards and reliability, and a learning culture correlate with these composites.

Areas for improvement identified in the survey results included communication openness, hospital management support for patient safety, staffing and work pace, communication about errors, and reporting patient safety events. While all achieved a positive score of over 50%, all 5 composites were below the international benchmark. Similar areas of improvement were found in previous studies, specifically, staffing and work pace, communication about errors, and reporting patient safety events. In addition, handoffs and transitions also needed improvement [21,22]. When we triangulate these results, with those from the GTT and AE, the overall results relate most to the three SC components of prioritising safety, reporting, and just culture.

4.1. Prioritising Safety

There is a significant difference between perceived Supervisor/Manager support for patient safety and Hospital management support despite both composites correlating with the Prioritising Safety component. This dichotomy may be explained by staff perceiving their local managers to be more involved in developing a good safety culture while perceiving managers more removed from them to be less involved in the unit's safety culture. While the hospital has an active quality and safety improvement directorate supporting over 20 programmes of work addressing key risks within the hospital, front-line staff may not be as intimately aware of these and other patient safety efforts managed and delivered by colleagues less closely connected with them in the hospital. These findings are similar to those from other national studies [33–35]. This is also highlighted by the WHO Global Patient Safety Action Plan and the Health Service Executive in Ireland Patient Safety Strategy emphasising the need to build leadership and management capacity at all levels of the health system to ultimately achieve more resilient systems [4,36].

4.2. Just Culture

The low positive score in certain composites of the HSOPSC may indicate a lack of psychological safety and trust of staff to be supported by management, prerequisites to a just culture. Psychological safety relates to how individuals perceive their work environment as being supportive of them being able to ask questions and express concerns [37]. A just culture refers to "an atmosphere of trust in which people are encouraged, even rewarded, for providing essential safety-related information—but in which they are also clear about where the line must be drawn between acceptable and unacceptable behaviour" [6].

When there is a lack of psychological safety staff are less likely to speak up or report errors in fear of blame, resulting in a widening of the gap between work-as-done by clinicians and work-as-imagined by managers, resulting in less resilient systems of care [38]. This has a significant impact on patient safety, preventing quality improvement as underlying problems are not identified, resulting in failures to prevent the recurrence of AEs [38]. This is a key area for system improvement that can be addressed by acknowledging fallibility, actively seeking and valuing staff input, and addressing any hierarchical concerns of staff [37,38]. This has been highlighted as a key focus nationally in Ireland, requiring a multifaceted approach involving all stakeholders, where behaviours that remove fear of reprisal if incidents are reported and build trust that errors are managed fairly are embedded from the top down [39].

4.3. Reporting Culture

These results suggest a reluctance to report harm and poor communication of errors [27]. This was further emphasised in the qualitative data, with themes arising around communication issues and poor reporting culture. The association between lower SC scores and lower incident reporting was also seen in previous studies using more than one method of analysis [21,22]. When it comes to AE reporting, some reduction in reporting levels may be attributable to the impact of the COVID-19 pandemic at the time. The ongoing COVID-19 pandemic has caused increased emotional distress, burnout, and staff turnover in healthcare, especially in ICUs [40,41]. This study was completed after several waves of COVID-19, and burnout and exhaustion experienced by staff may have contributed to reduced reporting and impacted the SC. Internationally, studies have shown there has been a reduction in reporting during COVID-19, estimated at 4.4% overall [23,42,43]. When examined in terms of category, the reduction was in "no harm" and "near miss" AEs, with little change in the number of "harm" events reported, which seems to be reflected in our study [23]. Various factors may have influenced this, such as increased workload, lower staffing levels, and time to report, and changed the perception of the importance of AE reporting, especially near misses and no-harm events [43]. The reduction in reporting may represent potential lost learning opportunities to improve patient safety during an unprecedented time [23]. The hospital's safety and risk management policies strongly encourage AE reporting in the case of harm or near miss, related or unrelated to the provision of care, regardless of the severity.

5. Conclusions

All seven components of SC need to be present to achieve a positive SC and have a lasting impact on patient safety [6,7]. This study demonstrates the importance of examining all the components of SC from different perspectives. While our triangulation sheds the most light on the components of prioritising safety, reporting, and just culture, it has shown that, when looked at from different perspectives, improvements are needed in all these areas. Some authors would argue that psychological safety, speaking up about safety, and a supporting just culture, which ensures we are not blamed for mistakes (but held to account when we do deliberate harm), are the most important building blocks of a positive SC (e.g., [37,38]).

Changing culture, and SC in particular, is an essential component of whole system change [44]. There are few case studies or reports of successful system change in healthcare, and there is a lack of agreement on "whole system change" [45]. To achieve improvements in patient safety, there first needs to be a shift towards a whole systems approach with a clear understanding of the goals of that system—patient safety must be a key goal of our healthcare system and perceived by all staff as a key priority for the organisation, as outlined in the WHO Global Patient Safety Action Plan [4,45]. A whole systems approach prioritising patient safety would then enable collaborative working to achieve sustained improvements in patient safety. Successful large-scale projects aiming to reduce harm in the ICU have been founded on creating a positive SC that meaningfully engages clinicians, patients, and families [46–48] and have adopted methodologies focused on strong system designs with goals of safety, high efficiency, and value [48]. The findings from this study have been presented to the ICU MDT and at fora across the hospital. A SC improvement plan has been put in place and learning from this study has contributed to ongoing system change for quality and safety improvement in the hospital.

Limitations and Future Research

There are some limitations to the study. Understanding SC is very difficult. To really achieve triangulation on the different components of SC as per the adaptation of the Reason model [7,8] would have required a much larger study. The triangulation of data in this study was achieved for three components of safety culture, which are priority, reporting, and just culture. As outlined by the WHO [4], the engagement of patients and families in the assessment of SC would likely have provided another aspect of assessment and should be considered for future, larger-scale studies. This is a one-time-point study with all data gathered within a four-week timeframe. It would have been beneficial to complete further chart reviews over a longer time period, although the charts reviewed were randomly selected as per Institute for Healthcare Improvement guidance, and reviewing additional charts may not have added anything of further significance to the study. As this study was completed after multiple COVID-19 waves, emotional distress, staff burnout, staff turnover, and changes in the work environment may have significantly impacted the findings from the study. This may have influenced the low response rate, despite attempts at recruiting more participants through staff meetings and email reminders, as outlined above.

Supplementary Materials: The following supporting information can be downloaded at: https://www.mdpi.com/article/10.3390/healthcare11233095/s1, Supplementary File S1: ICU adverse event trigger tool worksheet; Supplementary File S2: Hospital Survey on Patient Safety (Version 2.0).

Author Contributions: Conceptualization, E.L. and M.E.W.; methodology and data analysis E.L., M.E.W. and E.O. writing—original draft preparation, E.L.; writing—review and editing, E.L., M.E.W. and E.O. supervision, M.E.W. and E.O.; All authors have read and agreed to the published version of the manuscript.

Funding: This research was part of a higher education program (Masters in Human Factors in Patient Safety, RCSI) for which the main author (EL) received funding from St James's Hospital.

Institutional Review Board Statement: The study was conducted according to the guidelines of the Declaration of Helsinki, the hospital GDPR and data protection office, and approved by the St James's Hospital and Tallaght University Hospital Joint Ethics Committee (Reference no. 645 Approval Date: 25 January 2022).

Informed Consent Statement: Informed consent was obtained from all subjects involved in the study. All staff were invited to participate on a voluntary basis and a participant information leaflet (PIL) was sent to all staff along with the link for an online survey. As the survey was completed anonymously the Ethics Committee agreed informed consent was implied through completion of the survey. All data was unidentifiable and remained anonymous. This study was undertaken with hospital staff; no patients or their family/carers were involved.

Data Availability Statement: The data presented in this study are available on request from the corresponding author. The data are not publicly available due to the sensitivity of the topic.

Acknowledgments: The authors would like to thank all of the ICU staff who participated in the survey. The authors would like to acknowledge the help and support of staff in the Quality and Safety Improvement Directorate Patient Safety Office in reviewing AEs and colleagues in the Physiotherapy department for their help with the GTT chart review.

Conflicts of Interest: The authors declare no conflict of interest.

References

1. Bienassis, D.E.; Klazinga, N.S. *Developing International Benchmarks of Patient Safety Culture in Hospital Care: Findings of the OECD Patient Safety Culture Pilot Data Collection and Considerations for Future Work*; OECD Publishing: Paris, France, 2022.
2. Ward, M.E.; Vaughan, D. 3 Acknowledging and nurturing complementary leadership contributions. In *Distributed Leadership in Nursing and Healthcare: Theory, Evidence and Development*; Open University Press: Maidenhead, UK, 2021; Volume 29.
3. O'Donovan, R.; Ward, M.; De Brún, A.; Mcauliffe, E. Safety culture in health care teams: A narrative review of the literature. *J. Nurs. Manag.* **2019**, *27*, 871–883. [CrossRef] [PubMed]
4. World Health Organization. *Global Patient Safety Action Plan 2021–2030: Towards Eliminating Avoidable Harm in Healthcare*; World Health Organization: Geneva, Switzerland, 2021.

5. Cooper, M.D. Towards a model of safety culture. *Saf. Sci.* **2000**, *36*, 111–136. [CrossRef]
6. Reason, J. *Managing the Risks of Organizational Accidents*; Ashgate Publishing Limited: Hampshire, UK, 1997.
7. Wang, L.; Sun, R. A new safety culture measurement tool and its application. *Int. J. Saf. Secur. Eng.* **2014**, *4*, 77–86. [CrossRef]
8. Connolly, W.; Li, B.; Conroy, R.; Hickey, A.; Williams, D.J.; Rafter, N. National and Institutional Trends in Adverse Events Over Time: A Systematic Review and Meta-analysis of Longitudinal Retrospective Patient Record Review Studies. *J. Patient Saf.* **2021**, *17*, 141. [CrossRef]
9. Provonost, P.; Ravitz, A.; Stoll, R.; Kennedy, S. Transforming Patient Safety: A Sector-Wide Systems Approach. Report of the WISH Patient Safety Forum. 2015. Available online: https://wish.org.qa/wp-content/uploads/2021/08/017E.pdf (accessed on 12 July 2022).
10. World Health Organization. *WHO Patient Safety. WHO Patient Safety Research: Better Knowledge for Safer Care*; World Health Organization: Geneva, Switzerland, 2009.
11. Busse, R.; Klazinga, N.; Panteli, D.; Quentin, W. (Eds.) *Improving Healthcare Quality in Europe: Characteristics, Effectiveness and Implementation of Different Strategies*; Health Policy Series, No 53; European Observatory on Health Systems and Policies: Copenhagen, Denmark, 2019.
12. Chang, Y.; Mark, B. Effects of learning climate and registered nurse staffing on medication errors. *Nurs. Res.* **2011**, *60*, 32–39. [CrossRef]
13. Livorsi, D.; Knobloch, M.J.; Blue, L.A.; Swafford, K.; Maze, L.; Riggins, K.; Hayward, T.; Safdar, N. A rapid assessment of barriers and facilitators to safety culture in an intensive care unit. *Int. Nurs. Rev.* **2016**, *63*, 372–376. [CrossRef]
14. Rafter, N. *The Frequency and Nature of Adverse Events in Acute Irish Hospitals: The Irish National Adverse Events Study*; Royal College of Surgeons in Ireland: Dublin, Ireland, 2016.
15. Connolly, W.; Rafter, N.; Conroy, R.M.; Stuart, C.; Hickey, A.; Williams, D.J. The Irish National Adverse Event Study-2 (INAES-2): Longitudinal trends in adverse event rates in the Irish healthcare system. *BMJ Qual. Saf.* **2021**, *30*, 547–558. [CrossRef]
16. Waterson, P.; Carman, E.M.; Manser, T.; Hammer, A. Hospital Survey on Patient Safety Culture (HSPSC): A systematic review of the psychometric properties of 62 international studies. *BMJ Open* **2019**, *9*, e026896. [CrossRef]
17. Churruca, K.; Ellis, L.A.; Pomare, C.; Hogden, A.; Bierbaum, M.; Long, J.C.; Olekalns, A.; Braithwaite, J. Dimensions of safety culture: A systematic review of quantitative, qualitative and mixed methods for assessing safety culture in hospitals. *BMJ Open* **2021**, *11*, e043982. [CrossRef]
18. Tlili, M.A.; Aouicha, W.; Sahli, J.; Ben Cheikh, A.; Mtiraoui, A.; Ajmi, T.; Zedini, C.; Chelbi, S.; Ben Rejeb, M.; Mallouli, M. Assessing patient safety culture in 15 intensive care units: A mixed-methods study. *BMC Health Serv. Res.* **2022**, *22*, 274. [CrossRef]
19. Farzi, S.; Moladoost, A.; Bahrami, M.; Farzi, S.; Etminani, R. Patient Safety Culture in Intensive Care Units from the Perspective of Nurses: A Cross-Sectional Study. *Iran. J. Nurs. Midwifery Res.* **2017**, *22*, 372–376. [CrossRef] [PubMed]
20. Gomides, M.D.; de Souza Fontes, A.M.; Silveira, A.O.; Sadoyama, G. Patient safety culture in the intensive care unit: Cross-study. *J. Infect. Dev. Ctries.* **2019**, *13*, 496–503. [CrossRef] [PubMed]
21. Mardon, R.E.; Khanna, K.; Sorra, J.; Dyer, N.; Famolaro, T. Exploring relationships between hospital patient safety culture and adverse events. *J. Patient Saf.* **2010**, *6*, 226–232. [CrossRef] [PubMed]
22. Simons, P.A.; Houben, R.; Vlayen, A.; Hellings, J.; Pijls-Johannesma, M.; Marneffe, W.; Vandijck, D. Does lean management improve patient safety culture? An extensive evaluation of safety culture in a radiotherapy institute. *Eur. J. Oncol. Nurs.* **2015**, *19*, 29–37.
23. Denning, M.; Goh, E.T.; Scott, A.; Martin, G.; Markar, S.; Flott, K.; Mason, S.; Przybylowicz, J.; Almonte, M.; Clarke, J. What has been the impact of COVID-19 on safety culture? A case study from a large metropolitan healthcare trust. *Int. J. Environ. Res. Public Health* **2020**, *17*, 7034.
24. Granel-Giménez, N.; Palmieri, P.A.; Watson-Badia, C.E.; Gómez-Ibáñez, R.; Leyva-Moral, J.M.; Bernabeu-Tamayo, M.D. Patient Safety Culture in European Hospitals: A Comparative Mixed Methods Study. *Int. J. Environ. Res. Public Health* **2022**, *19*, 939. [CrossRef]
25. Thomas, A.; Lomas, J.P. Establishing the use of a safety attitudes questionnaire to assess the safety climate across a critical care network. *J. Intensive Care Soc.* **2018**, *19*, 219–225. [CrossRef]
26. Hibbert, P.D.; Molloy, C.J.; Hooper, T.D.; Wiles, L.K.; Runciman, W.B.; Lachman, P.; Muething, S.E.; Braithwaite, J. The application of the Global Trigger Tool: A systematic review. *Int. J. Qual. Health Care* **2016**, *28*, 640–649. [CrossRef]
27. Agency for Health Research and Quality. *Guidance for HSOPS 2.0 Content*; Agency for Health Research and Quality: Rockville, MD, USA, 2021. Available online: https://www.ahrq.gov/sites/default/files/wysiwyg/sops/surveys/hospital/AHRQ-Hospital-Survey-2.0-Users-Guide-5.26.2021.pdf (accessed on 7 April 2022).
28. Resar, R.K.; Rozich, J.D.; Simmonds, T.; Haraden, C.R. A trigger tool to identify adverse events in the intensive care unit. *Jt. Comm. J. Qual. Patient Saf.* **2006**, *32*, 585–590. [CrossRef]
29. Adler, L.; Denham, C.R.; Mckeever, M.; Purinton, R.; Guilloteau, F.; Moorhead, J.D.; Resar, R. Global trigger tool: Implementation basics. *J. Patient Saf.* **2008**, *4*, 245–249. [CrossRef]
30. Griffin, F.; Resar, R. *IHI Global Trigger Tool for Measuring Adverse Events*; IHI Innovation Series White Paper; Institute for Healthcare Improvement: Cambridge, MA, USA, 2009.

31. Sharma, A.; Minh Duc, N.T.; Luu Lam Thang, T.; Nam, N.H.; Ng, S.J.; Abbas, K.S.; Huy, N.T.; Marušić, A.; Paul, C.L.; Kwok, J.; et al. A Consensus-Based Checklist for Reporting of Survey Studies (CROSS). *J. Gen. Intern. Med.* **2021**, *36*, 3179–3187. [CrossRef] [PubMed]
32. Vaismoradi, M.; Jones, J.; Turunen, H.; Snelgrove, S. Theme development in qualitative content analysis and thematic analysis. *J. Nurs. Educ. Pr.* **2016**, *6*, 100. [CrossRef]
33. Relihan, E.; Glynn, S.; Daly, D.; Silke, B.; Ryder, S. Measuring and benchmarking safety culture: Application of the safety attitudes questionnaire to an acute medical admissions unit. *Ir. J. Med. Sci.* **2009**, *178*, 433–439. [CrossRef] [PubMed]
34. Dwyer, L.; Smith, A.; Mcdermott, R.; Breatnach, C.; El-Khuffash, A.; Corcoran, J. Staff Attitudes towards Patient Safety Culture and Working Conditions in an Irish Tertiary Neonatal Unit. 2018. Available online: https://www.lenus.ie/handle/10147/623433 (accessed on 10 June 2022).
35. Gleeson, L.L.; Tobin, L.; O'Brien, G.L.; Crowley, E.K.; Delaney, A.; O'Mahony, D.; Byrne, S. Safety culture in a major accredited Irish university teaching hospital: A mixed methods study using the safety attitudes questionnaire. *Ir. J. Med. Sci. (1971-)* **2020**, *189*, 1171–1178. [CrossRef] [PubMed]
36. Health Services Executive. *Patient Safety Strategy 2019–2024*; Health Services Executive: Dublin, Ireland, 2019.
37. Edmondson, A.C.; Higgins, M.; Singer, S.; Weiner, J. Understanding psychological safety in health care and education organizations: A comparative perspective. *Res. Hum. Dev.* **2016**, *13*, 65–83. [CrossRef]
38. Sujan, M.A.; Huang, H.; Biggerstaff, D. *Trust and Psychological Safety as Facilitators of Resilient Health Care: Working Across Boundaries*; CRC Press: Boca Raton, FL, USA, 2019.
39. Hughes, S. The Development of a Just Culture in the HSE, Health Service Executive, Dublin. 2022. Available online: https://www.hse.ie/eng/about/who/nqpsd/qps-incident-management/just-culture-overview.pdf (accessed on 10 October 2023).
40. Bradley, M.; Chahar, P. Burnout of healthcare providers during COVID-19. *Clevel. Clin. J. Med.* **2020**. [CrossRef] [PubMed]
41. Lasalvia, A.; Amaddeo, F.; Porru, S.; Carta, A.; Tardivo, S.; Bovo, C.; Ruggeri, M.; Bonetto, C. Levels of burn-out among healthcare workers during the COVID-19 pandemic and their associated factors: A cross-sectional study in a tertiary hospital of a highly burdened area of north-east Italy. *BMJ Open* **2021**, *11*, e045127. [CrossRef]
42. Zhang, X.; Sumathipala, M.; Zitnik, M. Population-scale patient safety data reveal inequalities in adverse events before and during COVID-19 pandemic. *medRxiv* **2021**. [CrossRef]
43. Pauletti, G.; Girotto, C.; De Luca, G.; Saieva, A.M. Incident reporting reduction during the COVID-19 pandemic in a tertiary Italian hospital: A retrospective analysis. *Int. J. Qual. Health Care* **2022**, *34*, mzab161. [CrossRef]
44. Mcnamara, M.; Ward, M.; Teeling, S.P. Making a Sustainable Difference to People, Processes and Systems: Whole-Systems Approaches to Process Improvement in Health Systems. *Int. J. Environ. Res. Public Health* **2023**, *20*, 5232. [CrossRef]
45. Ward, M.E.; Daly, A.; Mcnamara, M.; Garvey, S.; Teeling, S.P. A Case Study of a Whole System Approach to Improvement in an Acute Hospital Setting. *Int. J. Environ. Res. Public Health* **2022**, *19*, 1246. [CrossRef] [PubMed]
46. Sexton, J.B.; Berenholtz, S.M.; Goeschel, C.A.; Watson, S.R.; Holzmueller, C.G.; Thompson, D.A.; Hyzy, R.C.; Marsteller, J.A.; Schumacher, K.; Pronovost, P.J. Assessing and improving safety climate in a large cohort of intensive care units. *Crit. Care Med.* **2011**, *39*, 934–939. [CrossRef]
47. Thornton, K.C.; Schwarz, J.J.; Gross, A.K.; Anderson, W.G.; Liu, K.D.; Romig, M.C.; Schell-Chaple, H.; Pronovost, P.J.; Sapirstein, A.; Gropper, M.A. Preventing harm in the ICU—Building a culture of safety and engaging patients and families. *Crit. Care Med.* **2017**, *45*, 1531–1537. [CrossRef] [PubMed]
48. Dunstan, E.; Cook, J.L.; Coyer, F. Safety culture in intensive care internationally and in Australia: A narrative review of the literature. *Aust. Crit. Care* **2019**, *32*, 524–539. [CrossRef] [PubMed]

healthcare

MDPI

Article

Unpacking Perceptions on Patient Safety: A Study of Nursing Home Staff in Italy

Ilaria Tocco Tussardi [1,*], Stefano Tardivo [1], Maria Angela Mazzi [2], Michela Rimondini [2], Donatella Visentin [3], Isolde Martina Busch [2], Emanuele Torri [4] and Francesca Moretti [2]

1 Department of Diagnostics and Public Health, Section of Hygiene, University of Verona, 37134 Verona, Italy
2 Department of Neurosciences, Biomedicine and Movement Sciences, University of Verona, 37134 Verona, Italy
3 Department of Prevention, Healthcare Trust of the Autonomous Province of Trento, 38123 Trento, Italy
4 Clinical Governance Service, Healthcare Trust of the Autonomous Province of Trento, 38123 Trento, Italy
* Correspondence: ilaria.toccotussardi@univr.it

Abstract: Nursing homes (NHs) are crucial for de-hospitalization and addressing the needs of non-self-sufficient individuals with complex health issues. This study investigates the patient safety culture (PSC) in NHs within a northern Italian region, focusing on factor influencing overall safety perceptions and their contributions to subjective judgements of safety. A cross-sectional study was conducted on 25 NHs in the Autonomous Province of Trento. The Nursing Home Survey on Patient Safety Culture (NHSPSC) was utilized to assess PSC among NH staff. Multilevel linear regression and post hoc dominance analyses were conducted to investigate variabilities in PSC among staff and NHs and to assess the extent to which PSC dimensions explain overall perceptions of PS. Analysis of 1080 questionnaires (44% response rate) revealed heterogeneity in PSC across dimensions and NHs, with management support, organizational learning, and supervisor expectations significantly influencing overall safety perceptions. Despite some areas of concern, overall safety perceptions were satisfactory. However, the correlation between individual dimensions and overall ratings of safety was moderate, suggesting the need to enhance the maturity level of PSCs. Promoting a shift in PSC could enhance transparency, prioritize resident safety, empower nursing staff, and increase family satisfaction with care provided in NHs. The support provided by management to PSC appears essential to influence NH staff perceptions of PS.

Keywords: nursing homes; patient safety culture; Italy; long-term care; healthcare workers; safety perceptions

1. Introduction

Residential and semi-residential (day-care) facilities play an essential role in caring for the elderly, as they support de-hospitalization and meet the care needs of individuals who are not self-sufficient and/or are affected by complex health issues. In Italy, about 21 in every 1000 elderly individuals reside in nursing homes (NHs), with around 16 out of every 1000 residents being not self-sufficient [1]. Institutionalization rates increase with age, peaking at 76 per 1000 for those over 85 years old [1]. The COVID-19 pandemic has underscored the vulnerability of NHs, where the risk of care errors is notably high, leading to adverse effects on quality of life, morbidity, and mortality [2–6]. The heightened risk stems from various factors, including residents' multi-morbidity and multiple therapies and the necessity for interdisciplinary coordination, functional dependency, and cognitive impairment, all of which increase the likelihood of serious consequences from errors [2,7]. In addition, the care model of NHs is considerably different from the acute care and outpatient settings, with most of the direct care provided by nurses. Additionally, NHs constitute a real and often permanent living environment for residents, impacting the quality of life and the transmission of diseases [4]. These factors highlight NHs as a care system with unique safety concerns [2].

The promotion of patient safety culture (PSC) has become an internationally recognized priority [8,9], with extensive research conducted in some healthcare settings like hospitals, while NHs have received less attention. Moreover, empirical studies on PSC in NHs predominantly originate from North American contexts, with a scarcity of evidence from European nations, as emphasized by Gartshore et al. in a 2017 scoping review [10]. While some studies on PSC in NHs have been undertaken in Norway [11–13], further research is needed to identify barriers to safe care delivery and potential areas for enhancement. It is acknowledged that safety culture varies across countries, necessitating tailored evaluations to devise effective interventions [14–17].

Measuring PSC remains a contentious issue, given that the core of culture comprises intangible and implicit assumptions [18]. To address this, 'safety climate' (the perceived value placed on safety in an organization at a particular time point) has been proposed as a measurable correlate of safety culture, reflecting tangible characteristics through individuals' attitudes and perceptions [19]. In this article, we will use the term 'culture' (the values placed on safety and the extent to which people take personal responsibility for safety in an organization).

In recent years, various tools have been developed to measure PSC, with the Nursing Home Survey on Patient Safety Culture (NHSPSC) being recommended at the European level [20]. This questionnaire, developed by the Agency for Healthcare Research and Quality (AHRQ), has demonstrated good psychometric properties across different countries [21–24], though its validation in Italian had not been conducted yet.

Despite the usefulness of safety climate questionnaires in pinpointing areas for improvement, safety culture is multidimensional and influenced by staff culture, beliefs, values, and attitudes [25]. Understanding the predictive factors' interplay and their relative impacts on safety assessments is vital for prioritizing corrective interventions [26]. The study hypothesis is that each dimension of PSC can have a different influence on the formation of the overall judgment and overall perception of safety in the NH. Establishing the actual weight of each dimension in predicting patient safety is crucial for determining priority in implementing corrective interventions.

The aims of this study are:

1. To describe PSC in the NH setting within a northern Italian region;
2. To explore the factors influencing overall safety perceptions and identify their respective contributions to subjective judgments of safety.

2. Materials and Methods

2.1. Study Design and Setting

This cross-sectional study was conducted on a sample of NH workers in the Autonomous Province of Trento (APT), a region in north-eastern Italy. A single-stage cluster sampling method was used: initially, all NHs were invited to participate, and subsequently, all staff members of participating NHs, including non-clinical professionals such as support and administrative staff, were included in the sampling frame.

The APT features a unique Healthcare Local Trust responsible for providing care to nearly 550,000 residents both from urban and rural areas. NH care is delivered through the public system, with 55 NHs offering a total of 4600 beds dedicated to non-self-sufficient individuals requiring continuous medical treatment and healthcare assistance not feasible at home [27]. Most residents are elderly. Of these 55 NHs, 25 (45.4%) agreed to participate in this study, forming our cluster sample. The number of beds in these NHs ranged from 38 to 199 (with a mean of 94.7), totaling 2368 beds, of which 207 (9.6%) were private.

The Italian version of the NHSPSC was implemented to investigate PSC among NH staff. Details of the validation process are available in the Appendix A. This study adhered to the Strengthening the Reporting of Observational Studies in Epidemiology (STROBE) guidelines and the user's guide for the NHSPSC provided by the Agency for Healthcare Research and Quality (AHRQ) [28]. Detailed information on the materials and methods employed in this study has been previously published by our group [29].

The data collection took place between June 2018 and February 2019. Inclusion criteria were being a NH operator. In total, 2478 surveys were distributed and 1224 were returned (49.4%). Detailed information on data collection has been previously published by our group [29]. Staff categories were defined in accordance with the original version of the NHSPSC as follows: Staff Manager (including the administrator, medical director, director of nursing, and physicians due to their low numbers); Administrative Staff (including administrative assistants, admissions staff, billing personnel, secretaries, and human resources staff); Nurses; Direct Care Staff (encompassing nursing assistants/aides, healthcare technicians, and physical therapists); Support Staff (comprising personnel not directly involved in resident care, such as drivers, food service workers, dietary staff, housekeeping staff, laundry staff, and maintenance workers); and Other Providers (such as dietitians, nutritionists, occupational/speech/respiratory therapists, social workers, and psychologists).

2.2. Survey Instrument

The original version of the NHSPSC comprises four sections. Section 1 consists of 42 items that assess 12 different patient safety dimensions using a 5-point Likert scale. The Likert scale prompts respondents to indicate their level of agreement with safety statements (ranging from 1 for "Strongly Disagree" to 5 for "Strongly Agree") or with safety scenarios (ranging from 1 for "Never" to 5 for "Always"). Additionally, respondents have the option to select "Not Applicable/Don't Know". Dimension scores were calculated as the mean Likert score across all items within the dimension. The percentage of positive, negative, and missing answers (PPA, PNA, and PMA, respectively) for each survey item and dimension was computed, as described elsewhere [29]. Section 2 aims to provide an overall safety assessment by directly soliciting respondents' opinions on resident safety using a 5-point scale ranging from "Failing" to "Excellent". Respondents are also asked, "Would you suggest this NH as safe?" Section 3 comprises seven questions pertaining to respondents' professional roles in the nursing home. The final section allows respondents to provide personal perspectives on residents' care and safety [21].

2.3. Analyses

Descriptive statistics were used to summarize Likert scores for items and dimensions at both the respondent and NH levels. This dual perspective, which accounts for cluster sampling, assumes that respondents working in the same facility may be more similar to each other than to workers in different facilities since they share the same background/context and common habits. Thus, the research results can focus on differential interpretations, and their implications can be addressed on two distinct levels. Specifically, intraclass correlation (ICC) was computed for each dimension to quantify the impact of NH heterogeneity: values exceeding 0.05 indicate substantial variation between clusters and suggest a multilevel approach, accounting for the nested structure of the dataset. Furthermore, the relationship between NHSPSC dimensions and Overall rating (E2), both within and between NHs, was explored by computing the corresponding Pearson correlation coefficient.

A set of preliminary multilevel linear regressions was applied to select both the respondent features, considered here as covariates, and NHSPSC dimensions (predictors) that significantly influence the overall rating on RS (dependent variable), resulting in a parsimonious model. A post hoc dominance analysis was then employed on the final model to elucidate each predictor's relative contribution to the dependent variable in terms of the decomposition of the R2 fit index, so predictors accounting for larger proportions of variance were labelled as more important. Specifically, this technique estimated the nested regressions obtained by all possible combinations of the predictors, while the set of covariates was always included; it then calculated the Shapley value decomposition (the average marginal contribution of each predictor across all possible nested models) and ranked each selected predictor [30,31].

All analyses were performed using Stata software, version 18 (StataCorp. 2023. Stata Statistical Software: Release 18. College Station, TX, USA: StataCorp LLC.).

3. Results

Out of the 1224 received questionnaires, 144 were deemed incomplete or lacked information pertinent to the present study's outcome and were therefore excluded. Consequently, the analysis encompassed a sample of 1080 questionnaires (44% of those distributed), with response rates ranging from 18% to 82% across the 25 NHs. The characteristics of respondents are detailed in Table 1.

Table 1. Background characteristics of responders and NHs.

Responders (n = 1080)	**N (%)**
Staff category	
Direct Care Staff	675 (65)
Nurse	154 (15)
Other Provider	67 (6)
Staff Manager [1]	66 (6)
Support Staff	42 (4)
Administrative Staff	32 (3)
Job tenure, number of years	
<1	121 (12)
1–2	122 (12)
3–5	134 (13)
6–10	176 (17)
≥11	479 (46)
missing	48 (4)
Work hours per week, n	
<15	19 (2)
16–24	215 (21)
25–40	760 (73)
>40	49 (5)
Work directly with residents	
Yes	907 (87)
No	133 (13)
Nursing Homes (n = 25)	
Staff size, n	
≤30	6 (24)
31–60	13 (52)
61–90	4 (16)
≥91	2 (8)
Beds, n	
≤60	8 (32)
61–100	10 (40)
101–150	4 (16)
≥151	3 (12)

[1] Physicians were included among Staff Managers due to their low number (n = 2).

Mean scores for the 12 PSC dimensions are presented in Table 2. The distribution of PPA and PNA for each survey item and dimension can be found in Appendix A (refer to Table A1). The four dimensions with the highest mean scores (i.e., Feedback and Communication about mistakes, Handoffs, Overall Perceptions, and Supervisor Expectations and Actions Promoting Resident Safety, RS) attained mean scores ranging from 3.8 to 4, with PPAs between 68% and 76%. Conversely, the three dimensions with the lowest mean scores (Staffing, Non-punitive response to mistakes, and Management Support for RS) achieved values between 3 and 3.2, with PPAs ranging from 37.7% to 43%. Notably, for these three dimensions, 16 out of 25 NHs (64%), 12 out of 25 (48%), and 11 out of 25 (44%) attained mean scores equal to or less than 3 (further details can be found in Table A3 of the Appendix A).

Table 2. Descriptive of patient safety culture dimensions and staff evaluations on own NH's safety (n = 1080).

Dimensions	Mean	SD	NH min	NH max	ICC	95% CI
1. Teamwork within units	3.4	0.8	2.9	4.0	0.12	0.07; 0.22
2. Staffing	3.0	0.7	2.5	3.6	0.11	0.06; 0.19
3. Compliance with Procedures	3.6	0.8	3.1	4.3	0.11	0.06; 0.20
4. Training and Skills	3.5	0.7	2.7	4.3	0.17	0.10; 0.28
5. Non-punitive Response to Mistakes	3.1	0.8	2.5	3.8	0.12	0.06; 0.22
6. Handoffs	3.9	0.8	3.2	4.6	0.16	0.09; 0.27
7. Feedback and Communication about Incidents	4.0	0.8	3.4	4.5	0.13	0.07; 0.23
8. Communication Openness	3.4	0.8	2.9	3.9	0.11	0.06; 0.20
9. Supervisor Expectations and Actions Promoting RS	3.8	0.8	3.2	4.2	0.12	0.06; 0.21
10. Overall Perceptions of RS	3.9	0.7	3.4	4.5	0.17	0.10; 0.28
11. Management Support	3.2	1.0	2.5	3.8	0.20	0.11; 0.31
12. Organizational Learning	3.6	0.7	2.9	4.1	0.18	0.11; 0.29
Global assessment						
E1: Willingness to recommend own NH *	74%	44	36%	95%	0.18	0.10;0.30
E2: Overall rating on RS	3.3	0.9	2.4	3.9	0.17	0.10; 0.28

RS = Resident Safety; NH = Nursing Home. * Answering "yes" to the item: "I would tell friends this nursing home is safe".

Regarding the overall safety assessment collected in Section 2, 74.3% of respondents indicated they would tell friends that their NH is safe for their family (E1). The mean value of the overall rating ('Please give this nursing home an overall rating on resident safety'—E2) was 3.3. Specifically, 42% of respondents rated the level as 'Very Good/Excellent', 38% as 'Good', and 20% as 'Fair/Poor'.

The variance in scores between NHs was moderate across all dimensions (ICC range: 0.11–0.20; refer to Table 2), indicating the presence of heterogeneity among facilities. The dimension Management Support for Resident Safety exhibited the highest ICC value (ICC = 0.20), suggesting that NH characteristics can account for 20% of its variability. Overall, the contextual effect was significant (ICC > 0.05; the confidence intervals, in the last column, estimate the presence of a contextual effect in each dimension), supporting the decision to employ a multilevel approach in subsequent analyses. A detailed description of the results of the surveys on PSC, stratified by NH, is provided in Table A3.

Table 3 presents the results of the exploratory correlation analysis, disaggregated within NHs (above the diagonal) and between NHs (below the diagonal) to differentiate individual- and facility-level correlations. All 12 dimensions and the Overall rating E2 were considered. The between-NH coefficients among the 12 dimensions exhibited high values ranging from 0.61 (between Management Support for RS and Compliance with procedures) to 0.94 (between Supervisor Expectations and Actions Promoting RS and Feedback and Communication); the consistency among these measures supports the multidimensional nature of safety culture. The correlation coefficients between the Overall rating E2 and the 12 dimensions between NH (last row of Table 3) varied between 0.077 and 0.318, indicating only moderate relationships. In the Appendix A, the frequency distribution of Overall rating (E2) and the dimension Overall perceptions of resident safety (Dimension 10) is further explored (Figure A1). The score distribution revealed a tendency towards higher values of the Overall perceptions dimension across all scale points. This result was confirmed with the intra-rater approach with paired data; the value of weighted Cohen's kappa is 0.31 (95% CI: 0.28–0.34), indicating a low or fair agreement between measures by following Cohen's suggestions [32].

Table 3. Relationship between NHSPSC dimensions and Overall rating on RS: within (above diagonal) and between (below diagonal) NHs correlation matrix.

	1.	2	3	4	5	6	7	8	9	10	11	12	E2
1. Teamwork	-	0.444	0.428	0.501	0.526	0.419	0.516	0.533	0.538	0.488	0.514	0.545	0.422
2. Staffing	0.775	-	0.377	0.423	0.453	0.396	0.353	0.413	0.392	0.422	0.443	0.445	0.363
3. Compliance with Procedures	0.832	0.793	-	0.402	0.394	0.283	0.349	0.277	0.35	0.419	0.3	0.412	0.318
4. Training and Skills	0.762	0.724	0.695	-	0.416	0.433	0.463	0.424	0.447	0.499	0.477	0.507	0.411
5. Non-punitive Response to Mistakes	0.822	0.830	0.796	0.857	-	0.415	0.475	0.542	0.469	0.433	0.5	0.522	0.388
6. Handoffs	0.652	0.849	0.737	0.700	0.823	-	0.594	0.554	0.511	0.505	0.467	0.53	0.418
7. Feedback and Communication	0.824	0.784	0.836	0.779	0.871	0.882	-	0.597	0.608	0.552	0.535	0.646	0.438
8. Communication Openness	0.752	0.674	0.628	0.731	0.771	0.789	0.882	-	0.611	0.469	0.59	0.582	0.416
9. Supervisor Expectations and Actions Promoting RS	0.829	0.706	0.834	0.744	0.812	0.806	0.940	0.866	-	0.577	0.579	0.633	0.458
10. Overall Perceptions of RS	0.790	0.787	0.779	0.699	0.710	0.764	0.872	0.809	0.818	-	0.59	0.705	0.633
11. Management Support for RS	0.682	0.644	0.609	0.710	0.650	0.661	0.766	0.794	0.674	0.837	-	0.649	0.49
12. Organizational Learning	0.836	0.821	0.818	0.824	0.824	0.819	0.938	0.835	0.857	0.927	0.846	-	0.541
E2 Overall rating	0.194	−0.11	0.174	0.296	0.108	0.077	0.218	0.318	0.303	0.095	0.148	0.149	-

Regarding the second aim, Figure 1 illustrates the heterogeneity of the Overall rating among NHs.

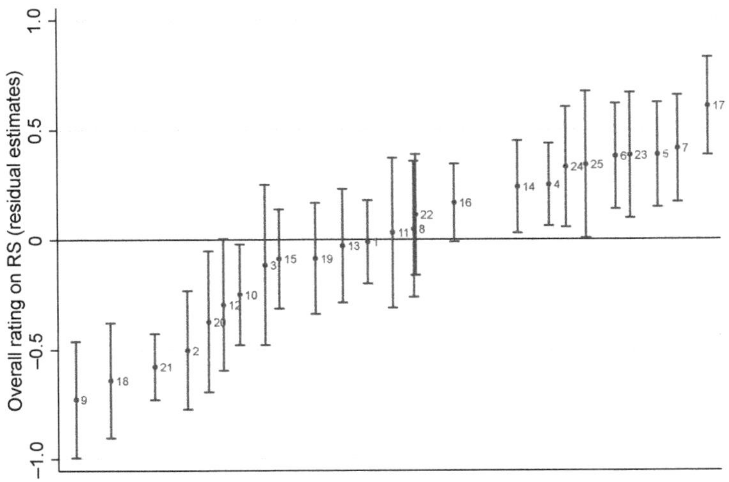

Figure 1. Caterpillar plot of Overall rating on RS, showing NHs residuals and 95% confidence intervals.

Table 4 presents the results of the multilevel final model and dominance analysis: seven dimensions significantly impacted the composition of the overall rating, accounting for the years of work experience of respondents, which emerged as the only covariate. The most influential factors affecting the overall judgment were Organizational Learning, Management Support for RS, and Supervisor expectations and actions promoting RS. The standardized dominance weighs ranged from 0.16 to 0.12, indicating a moderate differential impact.

Table 4. Multilevel model of overall rating on resident safety and dominance analysis.

Predictors	B (SE)	Std DW	Ranking
Organizational Learning	0.35 (0.05) **	0.1632	1
Management Support for RS	0.18 (0.03) **	0.1540	2
Supervisor Expectations and Actions Promoting RS	0.06 (0.04) *	0.1538	3
Handoffs	0.10 (0.03) **	0.1458	4
Teamwork	0.07 (0.03) *	0.1337	5
Training and Skills	0.09 (0.04) *	0.1275	6
Staffing	0.07 (0.03) *	0.1180	7
Work years (reference: 1 year+)	0.19 (0.06) **	0.0040	8
Pseudo R^2—level 1	0.42		
Pseudo R^2—level 2	0.76		

SE = standard error; * 0.01 < *p*-value < 0.05; ** *p*-value < 0.01; Std DW = Standardized Dominance Weights.

4. Discussion

In this cross-sectional study involving more than 1000 nursing NH providers, we aimed to highlight the safety perspectives of NH staff in Italy. The size of the sample, which represents almost half of all NHs in the study area, along with the satisfactory overall response rate, facilitated a valid portrayal of PSC among NH staff and identified areas for improvement within the NH setting.

The distribution of scores across dimensions exhibited heterogeneity, with a moderate portion of the variation (approximately between 10% and 20%) attributable to the facility level (i.e., affiliation with a specific NH). The observed heterogeneity between NHs suggests the need for strictly shared safety standards able to align expectations regarding safety behaviors. Moreover, the within and between correlations among dimensions suggest that individual factors beyond the facility level may also influence assessments. Indeed, the presence of safety subcultures within institutions is a well-documented phenomenon, although it has not been extensively studied in NHs, especially within the European region [10–13]. From a recent study conducted by our group, the presence of subcultures in Italian NHs appears to be associated with professional roles, as well as with overarching work-related factors such as seniority, working hours, shifts, and area of activity [29].

To prevent the development of subcultures and achieve successful clinical governance, alignment of leadership with workers is crucial [33–35]. Specifically, the support provided to safety culture via management is essential to consistently influence workers' perception of safety and overall satisfaction [36]. These observations are corroborated in our study by data from the dominance analysis, which emphasized how the three dimensions that most significantly affect overall judgment (Management Support for RS, Organizational Learning, and Supervisor Expectations and Actions Promoting RS) are all related to leadership.

From the responses to the individual items of Management Support for RS, a perception of management distance from frontline workers emerges, characterized by unsatisfactory receptivity to ideas and suggestions ("Management asks staff how the nursing home can improve resident safety" and "Management listens to staff ideas and suggestions to improve resident safety") and inadequate implementation of safety walk rounds ("Management often walks around the nursing home to check on resident care"). The high percentage of neutral responses in this dimension (ranging from 16.5% to 39%) supports the perception of hierarchical structures. Moreover, one out of four respondents indicated that management was not actively involved in decisions on how to improve resident safety. As previously noted, managers play a pivotal role in strengthening adaptive capacity within organizations, particularly when they are receptive to new perspectives and foster bottom-up initiatives [13,37]. Involving staff through a bottom-up approach has also been identified as a valuable strategy for ensuring resilient performance in addressing the challenges posed by the COVID-19 pandemic, as evidenced in a study by Ree et al. from 2022 [38]. Furthermore, safety walk rounds are an important and practical tool for enhancing PS within an institution [39]. However, to effectively implement them, it is imperative to proactively cultivate a safety culture to prevent them from being perceived as control measures, particularly in contexts where a punitive culture prevails.

The score for Organizational Learning was not entirely satisfactory, with suboptimal results observed for three out of four items. Specifically, difficulties emerged in implementing changes to improve patient safety ("It is easy to make changes to improve resident safety in this nursing home"). This result somewhat contradicts the positive assessment given to actions taken to improve safety ("This nursing home is always doing things to improve resident safety"), suggesting that despite some proactivity in certain contexts, actions do not seem to yield the perception of change. Ambiguity also arose from the results regarding the ability to learn from adverse events when they occur ("This nursing home lets the same mistakes happen again and again"—negatively worded item). The results on feedback and communication about incidents were satisfactory, indicating that if anything is lacking, it may be the ability to learn from errors.

To enhance the overall perception of safety, management should focus efforts on promoting a climate that facilitates changes and actions for the improvement of safety, as well as monitoring the results of these actions. Additionally, the process of learning from past errors should be promoted from a supervisor/management level so that personnel can perceive that care and attention are allocated to the prevention of adverse events. Organizational learning encourages the dissemination of best practices and evidence-based guidelines throughout the healthcare system, ensuring that lessons learned from past incidents are integrated into future practices. By prioritizing organizational learning, healthcare institutions can proactively mitigate risks, improve care processes, and ultimately enhance patient outcomes, thereby fostering a safer and more reliable healthcare environment [37].

The results concerning Supervisor Expectations and Actions Promoting RS underscore the significance of open communication in bolstering overall safety perceptions. Indeed, all items within the dimension are associated with transparent communication with staff and attentiveness to staff's work and suggestions. By fostering transparency, trust, collaboration, and shared decision-making, open communication not only mitigates the risk of medical errors but also enhances the overall quality of care [40]. Managers and supervisors must prioritize cultivating a culture of open communication where all stakeholders feel empowered to voice concerns, share information, and collaborate towards the common goal of providing safe and effective care to every patient.

The findings of the descriptive analysis unveiled notable discrepancies in evaluations across dimensions, particularly regarding Staffing, Non-punitive response to mistakes, and the previously discussed Management Support for RS. In fact, nearly half or more than half of the nursing homes recorded scores equal to or below 3 for these dimensions. At the individual level, the three dimensions attained PPAs around 40%, falling well below the satisfactory threshold of 60%, underscoring a pressing need for improvement. Similar outcomes were observed in prior studies [11–13] and are consistent with data from the 2019 AHRQ database, which provides benchmarking data from AHRQ survey users [41]. With the exception of Management Support for RS (66% PPA in the AHRQ database compared to 43% in our sample), the dimensions Staffing and Non-punitive response to mistakes exhibited the lowest scores, mirroring trends among the 191 nursing homes included in the AHRQ database. Specifically, Staffing emerged as the most critical area in our sample and demonstrated a comparable average PPA with the AHRQ database (i.e., 37.7% vs. 42%, respectively). For Non-punitive response to mistakes, the disparity between our sample and the reference database was more pronounced (i.e., 38.8% vs. 54%). It is noteworthy that the three dimensions with the highest scores in our sample (feedback and communication about incidents, Supervisor expectations and actions promoting RS, and Overall perceptions of RS) coincided with those scoring highest in the AHRQ database.

Regarding the Staffing dimension, the dominance analysis underscored its significance in shaping the final perception of safety. It is reasonable to assume that insufficient staffing levels and high turnover contribute to heavy workloads and difficulties in ensuring adequate patient safety, as indicated by low scores for items such as "We have enough staff to handle the workload", "Staff have to hurry because they have too much work to do", and "It is hard to keep residents safe here because so many staff quit their jobs". Additionally, the notable percentage of neutral and missing responses for individual items is noteworthy. While these responses may genuinely reflect a lack of clear opinion, they may also signify a reluctance to express negative perspectives. The literature highlights how high turnover is a prevalent issue in long-term care settings [42–44]. Turnover rates serve as useful indicators of NH quality and necessitate regular assessment and analysis to identify potential issues and provide necessary improvements [45].

Indeed, evidence suggests that high turnover may result in several adverse consequences for NH residents, such as an increased occurrence of physical restraint [45]. Moreover, it is likely that high turnover rates lead to a greater reliance on shortcuts during procedures, potentially compromising infection prevention and control, as evidenced during the COVID-19 pandemic [46]. Our results partially support this hypothesis, as the two items regarding compliance with procedures ("Staff use shortcuts to get their work done faster" and "To make work easier, staff often ignore procedures") garnered notable percentages of negative answers (respectively, 1 out of 4 and 1 out of 5 respondents agreed with these statements). Inadequate staffing may also have a detrimental impact on staff well-being, resulting in work overload and burnout [47,48]. Burnout, in turn, can affect both RS and the quality of care, creating a concerning cycle that underscores the importance of monitoring this indicator.

Regarding the Non-punitive response to mistakes dimension, the results highlighted the prevalence of a punitive safety culture among operators. To explain the deviation from the AHRQ database, we hypothesize that this is a particularly critical area in the Italian context. In general, an effective error-response mechanism necessitates that operators be adequately prepared to report mistakes, a responsibility that should be shouldered by management through targeted training and continuous feedback. Providing feedback is a crucial aspect of fostering a positive PSC. A study by Zwijnenberg et al. delved into healthcare professionals' perspectives on feedback from a PSC assessment [49]. The vast majority (84%) of respondents indicated that feedback partly or wholly stimulated actions to improve PSC, enabling staff to navigate the learning process through the mistakes themselves.

Specifically, regarding the Italian setting, a study by Tereanu et al. explored PSC in Italian territorial prevention facilities in Northern Italy [50]. The Non-punitive response to mistakes dimension scored a 39.5% PPA (38% among nurses and nurse aides) and ranked second lowest after Teamwork across units. The study also compared 10 composite measures with results from hospital settings (Italy and the US), health districts (Spain), and primary healthcare settings (Iran, Turkey). Italian hospitals scored lower (35%) than Italian territorial prevention facilities, which, in turn, scored lower than US hospitals (44%). Additionally, the study sample scored lower than the health district in Spain (42%). Overall, data from Italian settings indicate a generally low and less-developed safety culture in territorial facilities compared to hospitals, characterized by a persistent blame culture and under-reporting of incidents [51].

We also observed that staff expressed the need for more training ("Staff have enough training on how to handle difficult residents"), while simultaneously perceiving difficulties in implementing changes. This indicates the necessity of providing practical training through improvement projects that involve collaboration between staff and management to effectively introduce changes. However, despite the survey results, the dominance analysis indicates that this dimension does not significantly influence the overall perception of safety.

Furthermore, although the scores for some dimensions were not entirely positive, the Overall Perception of Resident Safety (dimension 10) achieved a satisfactory PPA of 76.4%, and the Global assessment section also showed positive scores. Moreover, the correlation between the twelve dimensions and the Overall rating (E2) was only moderate. These unexpected results suggest that item E2 provides additional information compared to that of individual dimensions, prompting reflections on the process of judgment generation by staff regarding their own NH. When tasked with assessing specific safety aspects, staff seem capable of identifying limitations. However, there appears to be a lack of ability to recognize these limitations as important threats to overall safety. Promoting an appropriate "preoccupation with failure", an essential element of a high-reliability organization, is crucial for improving safety culture. In this regard, sharing the results of the discrepancy between the scores of individual dimensions and the overall rating can help enhance this awareness.

In terms of actionable strategies that can be planned for implementing improvements, suggestions can be found in a practical guideline for PSC improvement promoted by the English NHS. The tool provides a comprehensive 'toolkit' to understand how to craft, create, and nurture a positive safety culture and offers a theoretical foundation for how to shift the culture. Among the key elements supporting a positive PSC are leadership, teamwork, communication, and organizational development [52]. A recent review by Taji et al. indicates that strategies for improving PSC in the hospital setting can be categorized into educational, simulation, team strategies, and comprehensive programs [53]. The review emphasizes that all types of strategies have a positive influence on PSC. Another recent review on strategies for improving PSC conducted by Mistri et al. highlights how education and training of healthcare professionals are crucial for strengthening systems and provides the descriptions of specific actions of improvement [54].

Strengths and Limitations

This study is part of the first attempt to assess PSC in the NH setting in Italy. It should be noted that this study was conducted on a single Italian region and on a limited number of NHs, and therefore the results may not be fully representative of the entire long-term care setting in Italy. The 25 NHs included in this study constituted a convenience sample, which could introduce potential research bias. The significant variation in the response rate of individual NHs may conceal additional biases related to the specific characteristics of the NH. Data were self-reported and possibly subject to social desirability biases. We have, however, limited the collection of socio-demographic information, which could influence the tendency to provide answers that are considered 'desirable'.

Additionally, the benchmarking comparison was performed using data from the AHRQ database, which primarily consists of information from North American NHs. Nevertheless, a notable strength of this study lies in the validation of the NHSPSC in Italian, providing a standardized tool for comparisons with other Italian settings, thereby enhancing the utility of benchmarking analyses.

In summary, this study serves as a foundational step for further exploration of PSC in the Italian NH context, through the development of a multi-centric study. Particularly, given the presumed association between PSC and actual safe care, further research is warranted to quantify this association with specific outcomes (such as falls, development of pressure ulcers, medication errors, adverse drug events, unplanned transfers to the hospital, etc.) within the country-specific NH context. Future research developments include the realization of a longitudinal study that could provide better insights into how improvements in management practices and organizational culture can influence PSC over time.

5. Conclusions

Measuring the safety culture of an organization is the primary and fundamental step towards instigating change and improvement. Ultimately, a shift in safety culture could cultivate an environment within NHs where transparency is esteemed, residents' safety is prioritized, nursing staff feel empowered, and families are satisfied with the care provided.

Author Contributions: Conceptualization, I.T.T., S.T., M.A.M., D.V., E.T. and F.M.; methodology, I.T.T., S.T., M.A.M., D.V., E.T. and F.M.; formal analysis, M.A.M.; investigation, I.T.T., S.T., D.V., E.T. and F.M.; data curation, I.T.T., M.A.M. and F.M.; writing—original draft preparation, I.T.T., M.A.M. and F.M.; writing—review and editing, I.T.T., S.T., M.A.M., M.R., I.M.B., E.T. and F.M.; visualization, M.R.; supervision, S.T., M.R., E.T. and F.M.; project administration, S.T., E.T. and F.M. All authors have read and agreed to the published version of the manuscript.

Funding: This research received no external funding.

Institutional Review Board Statement: This study was granted exemption from ethical approval by the Ethics Committee for Clinical Trials of the Autonomous Province of Trento (approval date: 8 June 2018).

Informed Consent Statement: Informed consent was obtained from all subjects involved in this study.

Data Availability Statement: The data presented in this study are available upon reasonable request to the corresponding author.

Conflicts of Interest: The authors declare no conflicts of interest.

Appendix A

Validation of the Italian Version of NHSPSC

The Italian version of the NHSPSC was developed following the seven steps outlined in the AHRQ translation guidelines [55]. A dedicated team, consisting of five researchers with fluency in English and diverse expertise, undertook the translation process and made cultural adaptations tailored to the Italian context. Specifically, the team comprised two researchers experienced in safety culture assessment and questionnaire translation (F.M. and I.T.T.), one expert in questionnaire validation methodology (M.A.M.), one with direct care experience in nursing homes (D.V.), and one specializing in accreditation processes (E.T.).

To ensure accuracy, the translated questionnaire was back translated into English for verification. Subsequently, a draft version was pre-tested with a focus group comprising seven NH staff members with varying professional backgrounds, including direct care, administrative, and support roles, to evaluate item comprehensibility, relevance, and clarity. A few suggestions for improvement were provided. The primary modification involved item B3 ("We have all the information we need when residents are transferred from hospital"), which was split into two items (B3a and B3b) based on the patient's transfer origin: hospitals/other nursing homes (item B3a: "We have all the information we need when residents are transferred from a hospital or another nursing home") or home (item B3b: "We have all the information we need when residents are transferred from home"). The final version of the questionnaire retained 43 items. Information pertaining to the additional item was integrated into the score of the 'Handoffs' dimension, ensuring that the survey's score range remained unaffected, as mean Likert scores were calculated accordingly.

The reliability of the Italian version showed good values, with Cronbach's alpha ranging from 0.58 to 0.89 (Table A2). Confirmatory factor analysis was conducted using the structural equation model approach to test how the original 12-factor solution fitted the Italian data. The estimated model showed acceptable fit values: RMSEA upper limit < 0.07 (RMSEA = 0.054, 90% confidence interval: 0.051—0.056); CFI > 0.90 (CFI = 0.912); TLI > 0.90 (TLI = 0.900); SRMR < 0.08 (SRMR = 0.056 relative/normed chi-square ratio—$\chi 2$/df—between 2 and 5 ($\chi 2$ = 2372.32, df = 794, $p < 0.01$)) [56].

Table A1. Frequencies of NHSPSC dimensions and items (n = 1080).

Dimension and Item	PPA (%)	PNA (%)	PMA (%)
1. Teamwork	**50.8**	**15.8**	**1.2**
A1. Staff in this nursing home treat each other with respect.	49.3	18.2	1.2
A2. Staff support one another in this nursing home.	55.2	13.0	0.7
A5. Staff feel like they are part of a team.	41.7	22.6	1.9
A9. When someone gets really busy in this nursing home, other staff help out.	56.9	9.3	1.2
2. Staffing	**37.7**	**37.7**	**2.8**
A3. We have enough staff to handle the workload.	21.7	52.9	1.3
A8. Staff have to hurry because they have too much work to do. (N)	16.9	58.6	0.8
A16. Residents' needs are met during shift changes.	70.3	8.9	4.5
A17. It is hard to keep residents safe here because so many staff quit their jobs. (N)	42.0	30.4	4.8
3. Compliance with Procedures	**60.2**	**15.9**	**2.7**
A4. Staff follow standard procedures to care for residents.	81.3	5.2	1.4
A6. Staff use shortcuts to get their work done faster. (N)	44.6	24.4	3.4
A14. To make work easier, staff often ignore procedures. (N)	54.6	18.2	3.4
4. Training and Skills	**58.9**	**14.9**	**2**
A7. Staff get the training they need in this nursing home.	70.5	9.9	1.1
A11. Staff have enough training on how to handle difficult residents.	45.7	24.4	2.1
A13. Staff understand the training they get in this nursing home.	60.5	10.5	2.8
5. Non-punitive Response to Mistakes	**38.8**	**27.1**	**5.3**
A10. Staff are blamed when a resident is harmed. (N)	32.2	26.0	7.5
A12. Staff are afraid to report their mistakes. (N)	39.6	28.3	3.3
A15. Staff are treated fairly when they make mistakes.	41.8	30.3	5.7
A18. Staff feel safe reporting their mistakes.	41.6	23.8	4.6
6. Handoffs	**67.5**	**7.9**	**3.4**
B1. Staff are told what they need to know before taking care of a resident for the first time.	69.4	8.3	2.7
B2. Staff are told right away when there is a change in a resident's care plan.	68.0	6.7	4.1
B3. We have all the information we need when residents are transferred from the hospital.	61.4	10.3	4.5
B3b. We have all the information we need when residents are transferred from their homes.	61.4	10.1	4.4
B10. Staff are given all the information they need to care for residents.	77.4	3.9	1.3
7. Feedback and Communication about Incidents	**74.4**	**7.1**	**2.2**
B4. When staff report something that could harm a resident, someone takes care of it.	71.9	8.0	3.3
B5. In this nursing home, we talk about ways to keep incidents from happening again.	70.2	10.1	1.9
B6. Staff tell someone if they see something that might harm a resident.	85.7	2.4	2.0
B8. In this nursing home, we discuss ways to keep residents safe from harm.	69.9	7.9	1.8
8. Communication Openness	**47.8**	**18**	**1.7**
B7. Staff ideas and suggestions are valued in this nursing home.	44.3	18.7	0.9
B9. Staff opinions are ignored in this nursing home. (N)	38.8	21.1	2.6
B11. It is easy for staff to speak up about problems in this nursing home.	60.3	14.2	1.6
9. Supervisor Expectations and Actions Promoting Resident Safety	**70.3**	**9**	**1.3**
C1. My supervisor listens to staff ideas and suggestions about resident safety.	69.8	7.7	1.0
C2. My supervisor says a good word to staff who follow the right procedures.	59.2	13.6	2.2
C3. My supervisor pays attention to safety problems in this nursing home.	81.9	5.8	0.7
10. Overall Perceptions of Resident Safety	**76.4**	**4.9**	**1**
D1. Residents are well cared for in this nursing home.	82.7	2.7	0.6
D6. This nursing home does a good job keeping residents safe.	71.7	6.9	1.4
D8. This nursing home is a safe place for residents.	74.8	5.1	0.9
11. Management Support for Resident Safety	**43**	**25.1**	**4.6**
D2. Management asks staff how the nursing home can improve resident safety.	46.3	22.0	4.4
D7. Management listens to staff ideas and suggestions to improve resident safety.	48.3	16.5	3.4
D9. Management often walks around the nursing home to check on resident care.	34.4	36.9	5.9

Table A1. *Cont.*

Dimension and Item	PPA (%)	PNA (%)	PMA (%)
12. Organizational Learning	**57**	**12.8**	**4.2**
D3. This nursing home lets the same mistakes happen again and again. (N)	58.9	14.2	4.5
D4. It is easy to make changes to improve resident safety in this nursing home.	44.2	19.7	3.2
D5. This nursing home is always doing things to improve resident safety.	65.6	8.2	2.3
D10. When this nursing home makes changes to improve resident safety, it checks to see if the changes worked.	59.3	9.0	6.9

Possible Likert score range is 1 to 5 points. Positive responses were considered 'Agree/Strongly Agree' or 'Most of the Time/Always' (score 4–5 on Likert scale) for positively worded items and, 'Disagree/Strongly Disagree' or 'Rarely/Never' (score 1–2 on Likert scale) for negatively worded items. The opposite applied when calculating the percentage of negative answers. PPA = percentage of positive answers (Likert 4–5). PNA = percentage of negative answers (Likert 1–2). PMA = percentage of missing answers. (N) = negatively worded items. The dimensions' scores consisted of the mean PPA, PNA, and PMA considering all items included in the dimension.

Table A2. Reliability analysis of the Italian NHSPSC and comparison with referral studies from North America and Europe.

Dimension	Item	Cronbach's Alpha		
		Italy	U.S. [15]	Norway [23]
1. Teamwork	A1, A2, A5, A9	0.87	0.79–0.83 *	0.79
2. Staffing	A3, A8, A16, A17	0.58	0.62	0.55
3. Compliance with Procedures	A4, A6, A14	0.70	-	0.58
4. Training and Skills	A7, A11, A13	0.68	-	0.67
5. Non-punitive Response to Mistakes	A10, A12, A15, A18	0.72	0.78	0.65
6. Handoffs	B1, B2, B3, B3b, B10	0.89	0.81	0.74
7. Feedback and Communication about Incidents	B4, B5, B6, B8	0.84	0.78	0.74
8. Communication Openness	B7, B9, B11	0.71	0.73	0.74
9. Supervisor Expectations and Actions Promoting Resident Safety	C1, C2, C3	0.84	0.79	0.84
10. Overall Perceptions of Resident Safety	D1, D6, D8	0.83	0.74	0.90 **
11. Management Support for Resident Safety	D2, D7, D9	0.85	0.79	0.90 **
12. Organizational Learning	D3, D4, D5, D10	0.72	0.71	0.90 **

* Teamwork across units: 0.79; teamwork within units: 0.83. ** Management and Organizational learning: the factor includes "overall perception of safety". "management support for patient safety", and "organizational learning".

Table A3. Descriptive of patient safety culture dimensions per NHs (SD).

NH	1	2	3	4	5	6	7	8	9	10	11	12
1	3.2 (0.8)	2.9 (0.6)	3.5 (0.7)	3.5 (0.7)	3.1 (0.7)	3.8 (0.7)	3.9 (0.8)	3.4 (0.7)	3.8 (0.8)	3.9 (0.7)	3.2 (0.9)	3.5 (0.6)
2	3.4 (0.9)	2.7 (0.7)	3.6 (0.8)	3.3 (0.7)	3.1 (0.7)	3.9 (0.6)	4.1 (0.8)	3.4 (0.8)	3.9 (0.6)	3.6 (0.7)	2.6 (1.0)	3.4 (0.7)
3	3.2 (0.7)	2.6 (0.5)	3.2 (0.4)	3.2 (0.6)	2.7 (0.4)	3.6 (0.8)	3.8 (0.8)	3.4 (0.8)	3.6 (0.8)	3.8 (0.7)	3.0 (0.9)	3.4 (0.6)
4	3.8 (0.7)	3.1 (0.5)	3.7 (0.6)	3.8 (0.6)	3.2 (0.7)	3.6 (0.7)	4.1 (0.8)	3.6 (0.7)	3.8 (0.7)	4.2 (0.5)	3.6 (0.8)	3.7 (0.6)
5	3.4 (0.7)	3.3 (0.6)	3.6 (0.6)	3.5 (0.7)	3.2 (0.7)	4.3 (0.6)	4.3 (0.7)	3.9 (0.8)	3.9 (0.8)	4.2 (0.5)	3.7 (0.9)	3.8 (0.6)
6	4.0 (0.8)	3.6 (0.8)	4.3 (0.7)	4.3 (0.7)	3.8 (0.9)	4.5 (0.6)	4.5 (0.6)	3.6 (0.7)	4.2 (0.6)	4.4 (0.6)	3.8 (1.0)	4.1 (0.6)
7	3.7 (0.6)	3.1 (0.7)	3.7 (0.6)	3.7 (0.6)	3.3 (0.6)	4.2 (0.6)	4.2 (0.5)	3.7 (0.7)	4.0 (0.6)	4.2 (0.5)	3.7 (0.7)	3.8 (0.5)
8	3.3 (0.5)	3.0 (0.6)	3.3 (0.7)	3.3 (0.6)	2.9 (0.6)	3.9 (0.7)	3.8 (0.7)	3.4 (0.7)	3.6 (0.6)	3.9 (0.5)	2.7 (0.6)	3.3 (0.6)
9	2.9 (0.8)	2.7 (0.6)	3.1 (0.7)	3.2 (0.7)	2.8 (0.8)	3.8 (0.7)	3.5 (0.9)	3.0 (0.7)	3.2 (1.0)	3.4 (0.7)	2.5 (1.0)	2.9 (0.8)
10	3.0 (0.8)	2.8 (0.6)	3.4 (0.8)	3.4 (0.6)	3.0 (0.5)	4.0 (0.9)	3.9 (0.9)	3.2 (0.8)	3.7 (0.8)	3.5 (0.8)	2.5 (0.8)	3.3 (0.8)
11	3.4 (0.8)	3.0 (0.6)	3.8 (0.7)	3.1 (0.8)	3.0 (0.7)	3.9 (0.7)	3.9 (0.7)	3.3 (0.7)	3.8 (0.7)	4.1 (0.5)	2.7 (1.0)	3.4 (0.7)
12	3.0 (1.0)	2.6 (0.5)	3.1 (0.7)	3.5 (0.7)	2.7 (0.6)	3.4 (0.7)	3.5 (0.8)	3.2 (0.5)	3.2 (0.6)	3.6 (0.6)	3.0 (0.7)	3.2 (0.6)
13	3.3 (0.7)	3.1 (0.6)	3.5 (0.7)	3.5 (0.7)	2.9 (0.7)	4.2 (0.8)	4.0 (0.7)	3.4 (0.8)	3.8 (0.7)	3.9 (0.7)	3.3 (0.7)	3.6 (0.6)
14	3.8 (0.8)	3.4 (0.9)	4.0 (0.7)	4.0 (0.7)	3.4 (0.9)	4.3 (0.8)	4.4 (0.6)	3.7 (0.8)	4.0 (0.6)	4.1 (0.6)	3.4 (1.1)	3.9 (0.6)
15	3.4 (0.6)	2.7 (0.6)	3.2 (0.7)	3.3 (0.7)	3.0 (0.6)	3.8 (0.8)	4.0 (0.7)	3.4 (0.7)	3.6 (0.6)	3.9 (0.6)	3.3 (0.7)	3.5 (0.5)

Table A3. *Cont.*

NH	1	2	3	4	5	6	7	8	9	10	11	12
16	3.5 (0.6)	2.8 (0.6)	3.7 (0.7)	3.8 (0.6)	3.2 (0.6)	4.0 (0.6)	4.3 (0.5)	3.6 (0.7)	4.2 (0.5)	4.1 (0.5)	3.2 (0.8)	3.7 (0.5)
17	3.6 (0.6)	3.2 (0.7)	3.8 (0.7)	3.9 (0.6)	3.2 (0.9)	4.4 (0.5)	4.4 (0.6)	3.6 (0.8)	4.1 (0.7)	4.5 (0.5)	3.7 (0.9)	4.1 (0.5)
18	3.0 (0.6)	2.8 (0.6)	3.1 (0.9)	3.4 (0.6)	2.9 (0.8)	3.5 (0.9)	3.6 (0.9)	2.9 (0.9)	3.3 (0.9)	3.4 (0.7)	2.7 (0.9)	3.1 (0.8)
19	3.1 (0.8)	3.0 (0.7)	3.4 (0.6)	3.1 (0.9)	3.0 (0.7)	4.0 (1.0)	4.0 (0.9)	3.0 (0.8)	3.4 (0.9)	4.0 (0.7)	3.0 (1.0)	3.5 (0.6)
20	2.9 (0.9)	2.5 (0.7)	3.4 (0.9)	2.7 (0.7)	2.2 (0.9)	3.2 (0.9)	3.4 (0.8)	2.7 (1.2)	3.2 (0.8)	3.5 (0.7)	2.9 (0.7)	3.0 (0.7)
21	3.4 (0.8)	2.7 (0.6)	3.5 (0.8)	3.3 (0.7)	3.0 (0.7)	3.6 (0.8)	3.7 (0.7)	3.1 (0.9)	3.6 (0.9)	3.5 (0.7)	2.6 (0.9)	3.2 (0.7)
22	3.2 (0.9)	2.9 (0.7)	3.6 (0.6)	3.8 (0.6)	3.2 (0.8)	4.2 (0.6)	4.3 (0.6)	3.8 (0.7)	3.9 (0.7)	4.2 (0.5)	3.8 (0.7)	3.7 (0.6)
23	3.6 (0.6)	3.2 (0.6)	4.0 (0.7)	3.9 (0.6)	3.5 (0.7)	4.6 (0.4)	4.5 (0.5)	3.9 (0.7)	4.2 (0.6)	4.2 (0.6)	3.7 (0.6)	3.8 (0.4)
24	3.5 (0.7)	3.0 (0.6)	3.5 (0.7)	3.7 (0.5)	3.1 (0.9)	4.0 (0.8)	4.2 (0.7)	3.6 (0.9)	3.9 (0.7)	4.1 (0.7)	3.5 (0.8)	3.6 (0.6)
25	3.8 (0.6)	3.1 (0.6)	3.7 (0.5)	3.7 (0.4)	3.5 (0.6)	4.3 (0.5)	4.3 (0.5)	3.8 (0.7)	4.1 (0.3)	4.3 (0.5)	3.8 (0.6)	3.8 (0.4)
Number of NHs scoring ≤3 for the dimension	5	16	0	1	12	0	0	4	0	0	11	2

Dimensions: 1. Teamwork, 2. Staffing, 3. Compliance with procedures, 4. Training and skills, 5. Non-punitive response to mistakes, 6. Handoff, 7. Feedback and communications about incidents, 8. Communication openness, 9. Supervisor Expectations and Actions Promoting Resident Safety, 10. Overall perceptions of resident safety, 11. Management Support for Resident Safety, 12. Organizational learning.

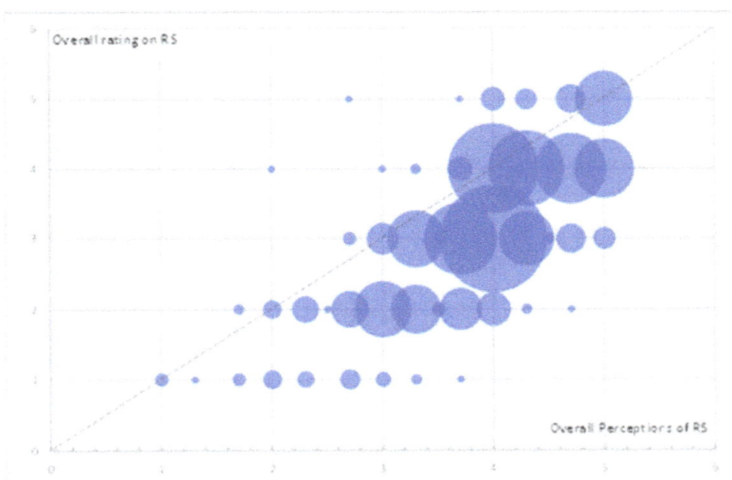

Figure A1. Bubble plot of "Overall rating on resident safety" (E2) against "Overall Perceptions of resident safety" (10th composite dimension): intra-rater comparison. Marker size is weighed by frequencies; the dotted line expresses agreement.

References

1. Ufficio Centrale di Statistica. *Annuario delle Statistiche Ufficiali del Ministero dell'Interno Ed. 2019*; Ministero dell'Interno: Rome, Italy, 2019. Available online: https://ucs.interno.gov.it/ucs/contenuti/Le_statistiche_ufficiali_del_ministero_dell_interno_ed._2019-10310230.htm (accessed on 10 July 2023).
2. Bonner, A.F.; Castle, N.G.; Perera, S.; Handler, S.M. Patient safety culture: A review of the nursing home literature and recommendations for practice. *Ann. Longterm Care* **2008**, *16*, 18–22. [PubMed]
3. Bor, A.; Matuz, M.; Csatordai, M.; Szalai, G.; Balint, A.; Benko, R.; Soós, G.; Dorò, P. Medication use and risk of falls among nursing home residents: A retrospective cohort study. *Int. J. Clin. Pharm.* **2017**, *39*, 408–415. [CrossRef] [PubMed]
4. Cazzoletti, L.; Zanolin, M.E.; Tocco Tussardi, I.; Alemayohu, M.A.; Zanetel, E.; Visentin, D.; Fabbri, L.; Giordani, M.; Ruscitti, G.; Benetollo, P.P.; et al. Risk Factors Associated with Nursing Home COVID-19 Outbreaks: A Retrospective Cohort Study. *Int. J. Environ. Res. Public Health* **2021**, *18*, 13175. [CrossRef] [PubMed]
5. Wisniewski, A.M.; Erdley, W.S.; Singh, R.; Servoss, T.J.; Naughton, B.J.; Singh, G. Assessment of safety attitudes in a skilled nursing facility. *Geriatr. Nurs.* **2007**, *28*, 126–136. [CrossRef]

6. Handler, S.M.; Wright, R.M.; Ruby, C.M.; Hanlon, J.T. Epidemiology of medication-related adverse events in nursing homes. *Am. J. Geriatr. Pharmacother.* **2006**, *4*, 264–272. [CrossRef] [PubMed]
7. Buljac-Samardzic, M.; van Wijngaarden, J.D.; Dekker-van Doorn, C.M. Safety culture in long-term care: A cross-sectional analysis of the Safety Attitudes Questionnaire in nursing and residential homes in the Netherlands. *BMJ Qual. Saf.* **2016**, *25*, 424–431. [CrossRef]
8. Castle, N.G.; Wagner, L.M.; Perera, S.; Ferguson, J.C.; Handler, S.M. Assessing resident safety culture in nursing homes: Using the nursing home survey on resident safety. *J. Patient Saf.* **2010**, *6*, 59–67. [CrossRef] [PubMed]
9. World Health Organization. Patient Safety. Available online: https://www.who.int/news-room/fact-sheets/detail/patient-safety (accessed on 10 July 2023).
10. Gartshore, E.; Waring, J.; Timmons, S. Patient safety culture in care homes for older people: A scoping review. *BMC Health Serv. Res.* **2017**, *17*, 752. [CrossRef]
11. Bondevik, G.T.; Hofoss, D.; Husebø, B.S.; Deilkås, E.C.T. Patient safety culture in Norwegian nursing homes. *BMC Health Serv. Res.* **2017**, *17*, 424. [CrossRef]
12. Cappelen, K.; Harris, A.; Aase, K. Variability in staff perceptions of patient safety culture in Norwegian nursing homes—A longitudinal cross-sectional study. *Saf. Health* **2018**, *4*, 9. [CrossRef]
13. Ree, E.; Wiig, S. Employees' perceptions of patient safety culture in Norwegian nursing homes and home care services. *BMC Health Serv. Res.* **2019**, *19*, 607. [CrossRef] [PubMed]
14. Castle, N.G.; Sonon, K.E. A culture of patient safety in nursing homes. *Qual. Saf. Health Care* **2006**, *15*, 405–408. [CrossRef] [PubMed]
15. Sorra, J.S.; Dyer, N. Multilevel psychometric properties of the AHRQ hospital survey on patient safety culture. *BMC Health Serv. Res.* **2010**, *10*, 199. [CrossRef]
16. Castle, N.G.; Wagner, L.M.; Ferguson, J.C.; Handler, S.M. Safety culture of nursing homes: Opinions of top managers. *Health Care Manag.* **2011**, *36*, 175–187. [CrossRef] [PubMed]
17. Fujita, S.; Seto, K.; Ito, S.; Wu, Y.; Huang, C.-C.; Hasegawa, T. The characteristics of patient safety culture in Japan, Taiwan and the United States. *BMC Health Serv. Res.* **2013**, *13*, 20. [CrossRef]
18. Schein, E.H. *Organizational Culture and Leadership*, 3rd ed.; Jossey-Bass: San Francisco, CA, USA, 2004.
19. Halligan, M.; Zecevic, A. Safety culture in healthcare: A review of concepts, dimensions, measures and progress. *BMJ Qual. Saf.* **2011**, *20*, 338–343. [CrossRef] [PubMed]
20. European Union Network for Patient Safety. A General Guide for Education and Training in Patient Safety. 2010. Available online: https://www.eu-patient.eu/globalassets/projects/eunetpas/guidelines_final_22-06-2010.pdf (accessed on 10 July 2023).
21. Agency for Healthcare Research and Quality. Nursing Home Survey on Patient Safety Culture. Available online: https://www.ahrq.gov/sops/surveys/nursing-home/index.html (accessed on 10 July 2023).
22. Zúñiga, F.; Schwappach, D.; De Geest, S.; Schwendimann, R. Psychometric properties of the Swiss version of the Nursing Home Survey on Patient Safety Culture. *Saf. Sci.* **2013**, *55*, 88–118. [CrossRef]
23. Cappelen, K.; Aase, K.; Storm, M.; Hetland, J.; Harris, A. Psychometric properties of the Nursing Home Survey on Patient Safety Culture in Norwegian nursing homes. *BMC Health Serv. Res.* **2016**, *16*, 446. [CrossRef]
24. Lin, S.Y.; Tseng, W.T.; Hsu, M.J.; Chiang, H.Y; Tseng, H.C. A psychometric evaluation of the Chinese version of the nursing home survey on patient safety culture. *J. Clin. Nurs.* **2017**, *26*, 4664–4674. [CrossRef]
25. Reason, J. Safety Paradoxes and Safety Culture. *Inj. Control. Saf. Promot.* **2000**, *7*, 3–14. [CrossRef]
26. Lee, S.E.; Dahinten, V.S. Using Dominance Analysis to Identify the Most Important Dimensions of Safety Culture for Predicting Patient Safety. *Int. J. Environ. Res. Public Health* **2021**, *18*, 7746. [CrossRef] [PubMed]
27. Provincia Autonoma di Trento. Trentino Salute. Demografia (Demografia e Situazione Socioeconomica). Available online: https://www.trentinosalute.net/Aree-tematiche/Osservatorio-per-la-salute/Profilo-di-salute/Profilo-di-salute-della-provincia-di-Trento-Aggiornamento-2019/01-Demografia-Demografia-e-situazione-socioeconomica (accessed on 7 February 2023).
28. Agency for Healthcare Research and Quality. Nursing Home Survey on Patient Safety Culture: User's Guide. Available online: https://www.ahrq.gov/sites/default/files/wysiwyg/sops/quality-patient-safety/patientsafetyculture/nursing-home/nursinghome-users-guide.pdf (accessed on 10 July 2023).
29. Tocco Tussardi, I.; Cazzoletti, L.; Zanoli, M.E.; Comini, A.; Visentin, D.; Torri, E.; Tardivo, S.; Moretti, F. Patient Safety Subcultures among Nursing Home Staff in Italy: A Cross-Sectional Study. *Healthcare* **2023**, *11*, 1962. [CrossRef] [PubMed]
30. Luchman, J.N. Determining relative importance in Stata using dominance analysis: Domin and domme. *Stata J.* **2021**, *21*, 510–538. [CrossRef]
31. Nathans, L.L.; Oswald, F.L.; Nimon, K.F. Interpreting Multiple Linear Regression: A Guidebook of Variable Importance. *Pract. Assess. Res. Eval.* **2012**, *17*, n9.
32. Cohen, J. Weighted kappa: Nominal scale agreement with provision for scaled disagreement or partial credit. *Psychol. Bull.* **1968**, *70*, 213–220. [CrossRef] [PubMed]
33. Degeling, P.; Sage, D.; Kennedy, J.; Perkins, R.; Zhang, K. A comparison of the impact of hospital reform on medical subcultures in some Australian and New Zealand hospitals. *Aust. Health Rev.* **1999**, *22*, 172–188. [CrossRef] [PubMed]

34. Horsburgh, M.; Perkins, R.; Coyle, B.; Degeling, P. The professional subcultures of students entering medicine, nursing and pharmacy programmes. *J. Interprof. Care* **2006**, *20*, 425–431. [CrossRef] [PubMed]
35. Lok, P.; Rhodes, J.; Westwood, B. The mediating role of organizational subcultures in health care organizations. *J. Health Org. Manag.* **2011**, *25*, 506–525. [CrossRef] [PubMed]
36. Lu, L.; Ko, Y.M.; Chen, H.Y.; Chueh, J.W.; Chen, P.Y.; Cooper, C.L. Patient Safety and Staff Well-Being: Organizational Culture as a Resource. *Int. J. Environ. Res. Public Health* **2022**, *19*, 3722. [CrossRef]
37. Hazy, J.K.; Uhl-Bien, M. Towards operationalizing complexity leadership: How generative, administrative and community-building leadership practices enact organizational outcomes. *Leadership* **2015**, *11*, 79–104. [CrossRef]
38. Ree, E.; Wiig, S.; Seljemo, C.; Wibe, T.; Lyng, H.B. Managers' strategies in handling the COVID-19 pandemic in Norwegian nursing homes and homecare services. *Leadersh. Health Serv.* **2022**, *36*, 200–218. [CrossRef] [PubMed]
39. Campbell, D.A., Jr.; Thompson, M. Patient safety rounds: Description of an inexpensive but important strategy to improve the safety culture. *Am. J. Med. Qual.* **2007**, *22*, 26–33. [CrossRef] [PubMed]
40. O'Daniel, M.; Rosenstein, A.H. Professional Communication and Team Collaboration. In *Patient Safety and Quality: An Evidence-Based Handbook for Nurses*; Hughes, R.G., Ed.; Agency for Healthcare Research and Quality: Rockville, MD, USA, 2008; Chapter 33.
41. Famolaro, T.; Yount, N.; Hare, R.; Thornton, S.; Fan, L.; Birch, R.; Sorra, J. *Nursing Home Survey on Patient Safety Culture 2019 User Database Report, Appendixes, Part II (Appendixes for AHRQ Publication No. 19-0027)*; Prepared by Westat, Rockville, MD, under contract No. HHSP233201500026I; Agency for Healthcare Research and Quality: Rockville, MD, USA, 2019.
42. Cho, E.; Lee, N.J.; Kim, E.Y.; Kim, S.; Lee, K.; Park, K.O.; Sung, Y.H. Nurse staffing level and overtime associated with patient safety, quality of care, and care left undone in hospitals: A cross-sectional study. *Int. J. Nurs. Stud.* **2016**, *60*, 263–271. [CrossRef]
43. McHugh, M.D.; Rochman, M.F.; Sloane, D.M.; Berg, R.A.; Mancini, M.E.; Nadkarni, V.M.; Merchant, R.M.; Aiken, L.H. American Heart Association's Get with The Guidelines-Resuscitation Investigators. Better Nurse Staffing and Nurse Work Environments Associated with Increased Survival of In-Hospital Cardiac Arrest Patients. *Med. Care* **2016**, *54*, 74–80. [CrossRef]
44. Kane, R.L.; Shamliyan, T.A.; Mueller, C.; Duval, S.; Wilt, T.J. The association of registered nurse staffing levels and patient out-comes: Systematic review and meta-analysis. *Med. Care* **2007**, *45*, 1195–1204. [CrossRef] [PubMed]
45. Castle, N.G.; Engberg, J. Staff turnover and quality of care in nursing homes. *Med. Care* **2005**, *43*, 616–626. [CrossRef] [PubMed]
46. Gandhi, A.; Yu, H.; Grabowski, D.C. High Nursing Staff Turnover in Nursing Homes Offers Important Quality Information. *Health Aff.* **2021**, *40*, 384–391. [CrossRef] [PubMed]
47. Leiter, M.P.; Maslach, C. A mediation model of job burnout. In *Research Companion to Organizational Health Psychology*; Antoniou, A.S.G., Cooper, C.L., Eds.; Edward Elgar: Cheltenham, UK, 2005; p. 544.e64.
48. Maslach, C. Understanding job burnout. In *Stress and Quality of Working Life: Current Perspectives in Occupational Health*; Rossi, A.M., Perrewe, P., Sauter, S., Eds.; Information Age Publishing: Greenwich, CT, USA, 2006; p. 37e51.
49. Zwijnenberg, N.C.; Hendriks, M.; Hoogervorst-Schilp, J.; Wagner, C. Healthcare professionals' views on feedback of a patient safety culture assessment. *BMC Health Serv. Res.* **2016**, *16*, 199. [CrossRef] [PubMed]
50. Tereanu, C.; Sampietro, G.; Sarnataro, F.; Mazzoleni, G.; Pesenti, B.; Sala, L.C.; Cecchetti, R.; Arvati, M.; Brioschi, D.; Viscardi, M.; et al. Exploring patient safety culture in preventive medicine settings: An experience from Northern Italy. *J. Prev. Med. Hyg.* **2017**, *58*, E121–E129.
51. Bodina, A.; Demarchi, A.; Castaldi, S. A web-based incident reporting system: A two years' experience in an Italian research and teaching hospital. *Ann. Ig.* **2014**, *26*, 219–225.
52. NHS England. Improving Patient Safety Culture—A Practical Guide. Available online: https://www.england.nhs.uk/long-read/improving-patient-safety-culture-a-practical-guide/ (accessed on 12 July 2024).
53. Taji, M.; Putra, K.R.; Ismail, D.D.S.L. Strategies to improving patient safety in hospitals. *Healthc. Low-Resour. Settings* **2023**, *11*, s1. [CrossRef]
54. Mistri, I.U.; Badge, A.; Shahu, S. Enhancing Patient Safety Culture in Hospitals. *Cureus* **2023**, *15*, e51159. [CrossRef]
55. Agency for Healthcare Research and Quality. Nursing Home Survey on Patient Safety Culture. Background and Information for Translators. Available online: https://www.ahrq.gov/sites/default/files/wysiwyg/professionals/quality-patient-safety/patientsafetyculture/nursing-home/resources/infotransNHSOPS.pdf (accessed on 19 June 2023).
56. Hooper, D.; Coughlan, J.; Mullen, M. Structural Equation Modelling: Guidelines for Determining Model Fit. *EJBRM* **2008**, *6*, 53–60.

healthcare

MDPI

Article

A SEIPS-Based Analysis to Understand Safety Culture During Postpartum Hemorrhage

Kaitlyn L. Hale-Lopez [1,*], Madelyn M. Saenz [1], Neelam Verma [2], Shruti Chakravarthy [2], Rebecca Ebert-Allen [3], William F. Bond [3] and Abigail R. Wooldridge [1,*]

[1] Department of Industrial and Enterprise Systems Engineering, Grainger College of Engineering, University of Illinois Urbana-Champaign, Urbana, IL 61801, USA
[2] Department of Obstetrics and Gynecology, University of Illinois College of Medicine Peoria, Peoria, IL 61805, USA
[3] Jump Simulation, a Collaboration of OSF Healthcare and the University of Illinois College of Medicine, Peoria, IL 61805, USA
* Correspondence: klh5@illinois.edu (K.L.H.-L.); arwool@illinois.edu (A.R.W.); Tel.: +1-217-300-8086 (A.R.W.)

Abstract: Background/Objectives: Maternal mortality occurs at alarming rates in the United States. In 2018, there were 17 maternal deaths for every 100,000 births—double that of other high-income countries, including France and Canada. Postpartum hemorrhage (i.e., excessive blood loss during delivery or within the 24 h following) is a leading cause of maternal mortality and is a treatable condition if identified and managed in a timely manner. One aspect of work that impacts patient care during postpartum hemorrhage is the safety culture. The safety culture is the beliefs, values, and norms shared by members of the organization that influence their actions and behaviors. In this study, we use the Systems Engineering Initiative for Patient Safety (SEIPS) model to understand and describe how the sociotechnical system shapes safety culture during postpartum hemorrhage. **Methods:** We conducted interviews and focus groups with 29 clinicians to describe the work system and the barriers and facilitators during postpartum hemorrhage. Then, we inductively categorized the barriers and facilitators into emergent properties of sociotechnical systems related to safety culture. **Results:** We identified 45 barriers and 158 facilitators into five emergent properties related to the safety culture (i.e., staffing, communication, organizational management and leadership, organizational processes, and teamwork). The participants identified more positive aspects than negative, suggesting that the safety culture positively influences their actions and behaviors. **Conclusions:** Our results indicate that safety culture could be improved by redesigning the work system to mitigate barriers related to staffing, communication, organizational management, and teamwork that hinder the safety culture.

Keywords: postpartum hemorrhage; Systems Engineering Initiative for Patient Safety; safety culture; sociotechnical systems

1. Introduction

Maternal mortality occurs at an alarming rate in the United States. In 2018, there were 17 maternal deaths for every 100,000 births—this ratio is double other high-income countries, including France and Canada [1,2]. A leading cause of maternal mortality is postpartum hemorrhage. Postpartum hemorrhage is when a patient has excessive blood loss; if within 24 h of delivery, it is considered primary postpartum hemorrhage, and if up to 12 weeks following delivery, it is considered secondary postpartum hemorrhage [3–5]. Postpartum hemorrhage can sometimes be prevented and, if not, can be better mitigated in treated if excessive blood loss is identified and interventions are initiated promptly [6, 7]. While variation exists in international guidelines on the management of PPH [8], care bundles that incorporate three or more evidence-based best practices can improve multiple postpartum hemorrhage outcomes [9], in particular the California Maternal Quality Care Collaborative (CMQCC) [10] and E-MOTIVE bundles [11]. Evidence-based best practices to intervene in postpartum hemorrhage include early prediction or warning systems (i.e., alerts), pharmacological treatments including uterotonics (e.g., oxytocin, prostaglandins) and coagulants (e.g., tranexamic acid, fibrinogen), intravenous crystalloids, uterine massage, intrauterine devices like the Bakri balloon and the Jada device, and surgical management (e.g., laparotomy, artery ligation, hysterectomy) [9,12–15]. Identifying that a patient is at increased risk for bleeding or is already having early bleeding allows clinicians to perform interventions to prepare for and stabilize the patient prior to a severe or catastrophic postpartum hemorrhage occurring. One aspect of work that impacts patient care during postpartum hemorrhage is the safety culture.

Before defining safety culture, and how it impacts postpartum hemorrhage care, let us first examine culture as a concept. Culture is composed of observable behaviors, artifacts, articulated values, and assumptions of groups of humans [16]—in short, cultures do not exist without humans, and some have argued that humans cannot exist without culture [17]. Discourse relating culture to work spans many levels; for example, how global and national culture influences work, cultures of specific professional groups [18], as well as cultures at the organizational level [19]. Organizational culture is the shared assumptions, values, and beliefs within an organization; newcomers to the organization are socialized through enculturation and taught that these are the proper ways to think, feel, and behave [20]. Some have argued that safety culture is a specific kind or facet of organizational culture [21]. While variation in definitions exist, there is consensus that safety culture consists of the beliefs, values, and norms shared by members of the organization that influence their actions and behaviors related to and/or in pursuit of safety [22–24]. Safety culture has been studied across industries [21]. In health care, safety culture, or patient safety culture, is widely acknowledged as crucial to improving safety for both patients and health care workers [25,26]—importantly, improving safety culture, and the safety of patients and workers, in health care requires a systems' perspective, rather than focusing on individuals in a piecemeal fashion [27,28].

In this paper, we present the argument that safety culture specifically, and any aspect of organizational culture in general, is part of the system in which workers perform their work. Our argument is rooted in human factors/ergonomics, which is, according to the International Ergonomics Association, "the scientific discipline concerned with the understanding of interactions among humans and other elements of a system, and the profession that applies theory, principles, data, and methods to design in order to optimize human well-being and overall system performance" [29]. More specifically, we draw on macroergonomics, the subdiscipline specializing in the design of organizations and work systems, with its strong theoretical grounding in sociotechnical systems (STS). STS theory arose from the Tavistock Institute after World War II, with a focus on improving work [30]. As indicated by the name, STS highlights that there are two subsystems: the social, consisting of people who sometimes work as teams, and the technical, including equipment, machines, tools, and technology, and these two subsystems interact within an internal environment that includes both the physical setting and organizational/managerial structure as well as the external environment [31,32]. The interactions between the people, technology, and environment shape how systems behave through emergent properties, which cannot be decomposed. Many approaches to understanding safety in STS have been described (see Carayon et al. [27] for a summary).

In this study, we use the work system model from macroergonomics [33–35], which is embedded in the Systems Engineering Initiative for Patient Safety (SEIPS) model [36–39]. These models posit that any work situation—where effortful activity is undertaken in pursuit of a goal, paid or unpaid—can be holistically described as composed of six work system elements (work system elements are italicized):

- The *team* of people who have their own unique skills, abilities, limitations, and characteristics.
- The *tasks* or goal-directed activities involved in pursuing the goal(s).
- The *tools and technologies* used in those tasks, including digital health technology, medical devices, paper and pencil, etc.
- The *physical environment* where the tasks are performed, which includes the physical layout, workstation design, noise, lighting, temperature, humidity, and air quality.
- The *organization* in which the work occurs, which includes both formal and informal organization, rules, procedures, management structures, climate, and culture.
- The *external environment* that includes rules, standards, and legislation outside of that particular organization as well as industry characteristics, like payment and reporting requirements in health care.

These work system elements interact and shape the processes involved in giving and receiving care (in care delivery settings) and activities that individuals take in pursuit of their own health in their homes and communities (e.g., patient work). These processes then result in outcomes for the patients, health care workers, and other formal and informal caregivers involved. The SEIPS model includes feedback loops, in which monitoring of system, process and outcome informs adjustment of the design of the work system—ideally, to bring about more positive outcomes. Importantly, culture is part of the organization's work system element: culture helps to shape how work processes unfold over time.

The interactions between system components (i.e., work system elements) result in emergent properties of the system, which can positively or negatively influence the workers, work, and outcomes—these emergent properties must be inferred from examining the system components as a whole [40–43]. Some of these interactions have been studied as work system barriers and facilitators—factors that hinder or help the performance of work and achievement of goals [44–47]. Work system barriers/facilitators can arise from characteristics of individual work system elements or the interaction of two or more work system elements involved proximally—in other words, those that are involved most closely and immediately to create that barrier/facilitator. Other work system elements can be involved distally, indirectly resulting in the barrier/facilitator. For example, organizational culture may specify a specific method for a clinician to complete a task, requiring the use of a poorly designed technology that is difficult to use, hindering a clinician from completing that task. In this case, the barrier is proximally related to the design of the tool and technology but distally related to the organization. Of course, with the systems view of SEIPS, at some point all work system elements will be distally involved, and developing methods to conceptualize, describe, and evaluate these multi-level interactions and 'system-ness' remains an ongoing opportunity [27,38,48,49], albeit with slow but steady progress [50–52].

In this study, we use the SEIPS model [36–38] to investigate and describe how the sociotechnical system shapes safety culture in postpartum hemorrhage in an academic tertiary medical center. Given our focus on safety culture, we are particularly interested in how other elements of the work system interact with the organization's work system element to impact culture.

2. Materials and Methods

This qualitative study is part of a larger project to design solutions to support the anticipation, detection, and response to maternal hemorrhage in prepartum, intrapartum, and postpartum care, aiming to ultimately reduce hemorrhage occurrence. This study is a secondary analysis of interview data [53]. The Institutional Review Board at Peoria determined that this study did not meet the definition of human subjects research.

2.1. Setting and Sample

The setting for this study is an obstetrics and gynecology (OB/GYN) department at an academic tertiary medical center in the Midwestern United States. The department staff includes 10 attending obstetrician physicians and obstetricians-in-training (i.e., resident physicians) each, 112 nurses, nine certified surgical technologists (CSTs) and 10 patient care technicians (PCTs). The year preceding data collection, delivery data at the participating medical center included 2259 deliveries and 261 hemorrhages (i.e., a hemorrhage rate of 11.6%). In these data, hemorrhages were defined as deliveries that were either coded as a hemorrhage and/or in which the patient had quantitative blood loss of >1000 mL (either or both of the previous) and that the patient received hemorrhage mitigation medications, underwent procedures, received transfusions, or had a predefined change in hematocrit. Hemorrhage procedures included uterine artery embolization, B-Lynch procedure, O'Leary stitch or uterine artery ligation, balloon compression (e.g., Bakri balloon), negative pressure system use (e.g., Jada device), suction dilation and curettage, or hysterectomy. Predefined changes in hematocrit included critically low values or significant change from baseline at admission for labor and delivery within 48 h of delivery.

We recruited 29 participants for this study, including five attending obstetricians, 11 obstetricians-in-training, 10 nurses, two CSTs, and one PCT between September and December 2023. The length of the experience of participants is shown in Table 1. We recruited participants in person and did not offer any incentive for participation. Participation was voluntary.

Table 1. Duration of the experience of participants in positions responding to postpartum hemorrhage.

Role	Number of Participants (n)	Average Experience (Years)	Range of Experience (Years)
Attending Obstetricians	5	8.8	2–18
Obstetricians-In-Training	11	1.86	0.5–3.5
Nurses	10	8.90	1–18
Certified Surgical Technologists	2	11.75	3.5–20
Patient Care Technicians	1	41	41

2.2. Data Collection Methods

We conducted semi-structured interviews in this study to allow follow-up probing for detailed responses [54]. The nurses, CSTs, and PCT were interviewed individually—due to scheduling constraints, the obstetricians and obstetricians-in-training were either interviewed individually or in small groups, separated by role.

Two researchers who were not affiliated with the OB/GYN department and thus did not have any authority over the participants led the interviews using an interview guide (the *Maternal Hemorrhage Interview Guide* is available at https://hfss.ise.illinois.edu/tools/, accessed on 17 February 2025). The questions included background information about the participant, the process and workflow of managing a postpartum hemorrhage across four phases of care, with probing questions about all elements of the work system, work system barriers and facilitators, and team formation and teamwork. One interviewer led each interview, while the other managed the logistics, kept time and took notes.

The interviews were conducted in person or via Zoom [55] and lasted an average of 39 min (total 12 h and 4 min). They were audio-recorded and transcribed.

2.3. Data Analysis Methods

The interview transcripts were reviewed for accuracy, and identifying details were removed. We uploaded each transcript to Dedoose (version 9.0.107) [56], a software used to manage qualitative and mixed methods analysis. As previously reported, we first performed a work system analysis and an inductive content analysis of the transcripts to identify all work system barriers and facilitators. Two researchers participated in the work system and barrier/facilitator analyses to enhance rigor; these results have been reported and identified 753 barriers/facilitators that were grouped into thirteen related groups: role ambiguity, anticipation, physical environment, staffing, resources/equipment, tools and technology, communication, coordination, cooperation, tacit knowledge, time pressure, leadership, and training [53].

In the current analysis, two researchers reviewed all individual barriers and facilitators to identify those related to safety culture. The barrier or facilitator was determined to be related to the safety culture if it reflected how organizational characteristics, such as the team culture, rules or processes, and management or leadership, influenced patient safety. We then inductively categorized those into broader dimensions and identified which work system element (or interaction between multiple elements) created those barriers or facilitators to positive safety culture.

We took special care to ensure rigor in this qualitative study [57]. We performed member checking to ensure credibility, clearly documented the context and methods to enhance transferability, and archived the iterations of our data analysis to enhance the dependability of our study [57,58]. Involving two researchers enhanced the credibility and confirmability of our work [57].

3. Results

We inductively categorized the 45 barriers and 158 facilitators into five emergent properties related to the safety culture (i.e., staffing, communication, organizational management and leadership, organizational processes, and teamwork). Figure 1 depicts the number of work system barriers and facilitators related to each emergent property, while Table 2 lists examples of barriers and facilitators.

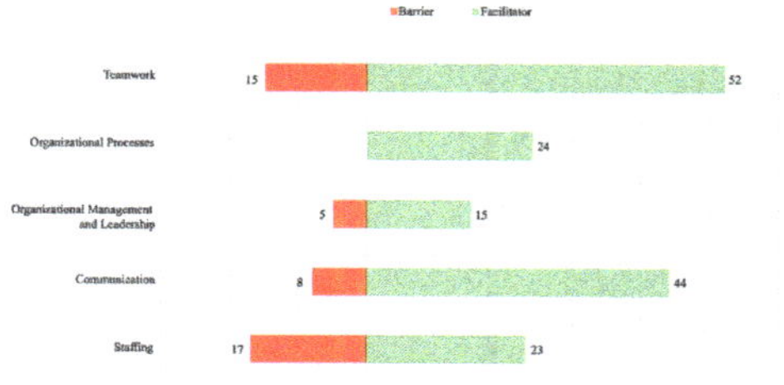

Figure 1. Count of work system barriers and facilitators by emergent property.

Table 2. Examples of barriers and facilitators in each emergent property.

Emergent Property	Proximally Involved Work System Element(s) *						Example
	Tm	T	TT	O	PE	EE	
Staffing	X	X		X			Barrier: *"I would say on the days when we are short-staffed. Everybody, it's almost like they have tunnel vision. They're so busy doing their own job that it's, you're, you're so busy. You're not seeing the full picture. Um, and it's very hard to work together because you just, like I got to get my job done, I got to get my stuff done."* (Labor and Delivery RN) Facilitator: *"Usually multiple nurses will respond as well, including like the charge nurse if it's becoming serious enough. So we have lots of hands, lots of help."* (Resident Physician)
Communication		X		X			Barrier: *"I think sometimes people just get flustered in emergency situations and it's hard to, for everyone to communicate."* (Labor and Delivery RN) Facilitator: *"I think, um, everyone is like comfortable with each other for the most part and is, feels comfortable like communicating concerns."* (Labor and Delivery RN)
Organizational Management and Leadership	X			X			Barrier: *"I'm always happy to be working with a nurse that has, years and years more experience than I do. I always feel more confident that way. Um, so it's generally a positive thing...I think that, um, it's something that [residents must learn], is how to navigate that. Because, um, you know, if they, for example, disagree with you on something, what do you do next?"* (Attending Physician) Facilitator: *"I think that there is a recognition that this is important. So we have regular mandated simulation days at least once a year regarding about, postpartum hemorrhage and what to do, and that's required for all attendings, residents and nursing staff and patient care techs. So once a year we do go to those and they focus on keeping that up to date, up to date. And we address also any hemorrhage incidents often in our QA committee. So we have a QA committee that reviews cases and if there's any significant findings, we address them and we talk about them there."* (Labor and Delivery RN)
Organizational Processes		X		X			Barrier: None. Facilitator: *"I mean there are like policies and procedures so that you can recognize it early and follow and follow the right algorithm to make the bleeding stop. Is anybody going to pull it off the computer at that particular moment? No, we just kind of know that A, B, and C are happening and we need to go...We need to address all of these and maybe go to D. And I mean, there's, I think the hemorrhage policy is posted places."* (Labor and Delivery RN)
Teamwork	X			X			Barrier: *"Well, it (the culture) would depend on, um, who was what we call the doc in the box. Um, that is like, or like laborist is what they call them. Um, there has to be somebody over on labor 24/7. So it would just depend on who was on that day. Um, you know, their demeanor, how they come in, um, somebody might be a little bit more high strung. Somebody might be a little bit more chill coming in, you know? Um, I think that depends. You know who's there, then the residents would come in, and again, it depends on personalities, you know who's coming in. And then also the labor nurses, they pretty much come in and just kind of take over, you know, everything but that's their cup of tea, you know. So, I think it just depends on more personalities."* (Certified Surgical Technologist) Facilitator: *"[We] oftentimes are working in very close-knit situations and we have each other's back and, um, take care of each other...We kind of have the opinion that all the patients on the floor are all of our patients and we just kind of help each other, especially like during emergencies and things like that."* (Labor and Delivery RN)

* Note: Tm = team, T = tasks, TT = tools and technology, O = organization, PE = physical environment, EE = external environment.

3.1. Staffing

Staffing refers to the availability of adequate and appropriate staff to manage the workload during postpartum hemorrhage events without feeling rushed (adapted from [22,59]).

The proximally involved work system elements are organization, team, and tasks, as the organizational management determines the number of staff members assigned to complete tasks each shift. This emergent property was mentioned in 17 barriers and 23 facilitators.

In 16 barriers, participants described that it is challenging to complete patient care tasks promptly when the unit is short-staffed. In the remaining barrier, a participant stated that when working with team members who are inexperienced in responding to postpartum hemorrhage events, the more experienced team members have to assume multiple roles to ensure the patient is safe.

In 15 facilitators, participants noted that when adequate staff is present, they can proactively assess the patient for symptoms of postpartum hemorrhage and perform patient care tasks promptly. In five facilitators, participants mentioned that an attending physician or resident physician is frequently available to support patient tasks, enabling timely patient care. In three facilitators, participants stated that when the unit is short-staffed, clinicians from other teams, such as the maternal-fetal transport team, can be reassigned to the labor and delivery unit.

3.2. Communication

Communication refers to factors that impact open and closed-loop communication about errors, preventing errors, or ensuring patient safety during postpartum hemorrhage events (adapted from [22,60]). The proximally involved work system elements are tasks and organization. The tasks element is proximally related, as communication, or lack thereof, impacts the patient care tasks performed during postpartum hemorrhage events. The organization element is proximally related, as the organizational culture may impact whether clinicians communicate openly to prevent errors and understand how errors occur. This emergent property was mentioned in eight barriers and 44 facilitators.

In seven barriers, participants stated that there is commonly a lack of communication between team members during postpartum hemorrhage response. They cited reasons such as clinicians being flustered during an emergency and physicians not being physically present in the labor and delivery unit. In the remaining barrier, a participant described how when there are varying perceptions about the hemorrhage risk level, they feel they must convince their teammates of their patient safety concerns.

In 27 facilitators, participants stated that they feel encouraged and comfortable speaking up when they have a patient safety concern and that they think their teammates are sharing pertinent information. Seven facilitators were related to participants using closed-loop communication during postpartum hemorrhage events. In six facilitators, participants stated that having resident physicians as teammates facilitates communication since they frequently ask questions or communicate their decision-making process. The remaining four facilitators were related to the use of technology, specifically pagers, to communicate that help is needed for an ongoing hemorrhage situation.

3.3. Organizational Management and Leadership

This property refers to how organizational management and leadership impact patient safety during postpartum hemorrhage events (adapted from [22,39]). The proximally involved work systems elements are organization and team, as organizational management and the leader of the team may influence patient safety, such as commitment to patient safety or collaboration between interdisciplinary departments. This emergent property was mentioned in five barriers and 15 facilitators.

In all five barriers, participants stated that the leadership of the team negatively impacts patient safety, as poor leadership causes a high-anxiety situation and makes it difficult to share their clinical opinion. In 11 facilitators, participants mentioned that a leader with prior experience, good communication skills, and a calm presence is helpful during postpartum hemorrhage events. The remaining four facilitators were related to how organizational leadership promotes patient safety during postpartum hemorrhage events. Participants stated that the organizational leadership mandated annual training for all team members to ensure they were aware of best practices and established a quality assurance committee to review cases of postpartum hemorrhage to identify possible improvements in patient safety.

3.4. Organizational Processes

This property refers to how the organizational rules, processes, and procedures impact patient safety during postpartum hemorrhage events (adapted from [22,39]). The proximally involved work system elements are tasks and organization. The tasks element is proximally involved as the organizational processes directly impact which tasks are performed and the order in which the tasks are performed. The organization element is proximally involved as these rules, processes, and procedures are set at the organizational level. This emergent property was not mentioned in any barriers. However, it was mentioned in 24 facilitators.

In 18 facilitators, participants mentioned that they follow a general postpartum hemorrhage management process, outlined by the organization, that follows best practices published by the American College of Obstetricians and Gynecologists. The remaining six facilitators were related to the organizational process of performing a retrospective on postpartum hemorrhage events. During these retrospectives, clinicians are encouraged to discuss what occurred during postpartum hemorrhage management and identify areas of improvement.

3.5. Teamwork

Teamwork refers to how the organizational culture and climate impact the willingness of each clinician to work together during postpartum hemorrhage events (adapted from [22,60]). The proximally involved work system elements are team and organization. The team element is proximally involved since members must be willing, or want to, cooperate within the team. The organization element is proximally involved as the organizational culture and climate impact teamwork. This emergent property was mentioned in 15 barriers and 52 facilitators.

In ten barriers, participants stated that the personality of their team members may negatively impact teamwork during postpartum hemorrhage events. Some participants said that they sometimes avoid voicing concerns about patient safety as it sometimes creates tension between team members. Relatedly, in three barriers, participants mentioned that they often feel burnt out from the high demands experienced during postpartum hemorrhage management, which may negatively impact teamwork. In the remaining two barriers, participants mentioned that teamwork is negatively affected by the prioritization of charting over patient care tasks and a perceived lack of support for clinical roles such as surgical technicians.

In 52 facilitators, participants described their teammates as helpful, respectful, knowledgeable, and collaborative. They said their teammates recognize the seriousness of postpartum hemorrhage and are willing to help one another, regardless of their workload. Additionally, participants mentioned that the organizational culture supported their willingness to ask for help.

4. Discussion

In this study, we identified five emergent properties that contain 158 facilitators and 45 barriers related to safety culture (i.e., staffing, communication, organizational management and leadership, organizational processes, and teamwork). Our findings provide insight into how the sociotechnical system is related to safety culture, specifically during postpartum hemorrhage; unsurprisingly, given our focus on safety culture, the organization work system element was focal.

4.1. Proximally Involved Work System Elements

The five emergent properties were proximally related to three of the six work system elements. As described in the methods, a proximally involved work system element is the element (or interaction between multiple work system elements) that created the work system barrier or facilitator [38]. The team, tasks, and organization elements directly impact the safety culture. As highlighted previously, the organization element was proximally related to the five emergent properties. In comparison, the team element was related to one, and the tasks element was related to two properties. Considering our original definition of safety culture as the beliefs, values, and norms shared by members of the organization that influence their actions and behaviors related to and/or in pursuit of safety [22–24], this is unsurprising. The *organization* element includes the culture of the organization—as mentioned previously, safety culture is a specific aspect of the culture of an organization. The behaviors of people—the things they do—often are performed as part of the tasks the people complete in the organization, hence the relationship to the *task* element. Finally, the team is the people who have their own experiences and characteristics that also relate to beliefs and values [39,61]. In our study, the physical environment, external environment, and tools and technologies elements did not directly impact the safety culture involved in the care of postpartum hemorrhage. However, we would argue that these are distally related to culture and may emerge in future studies. For example, what an organization values—distinctly part of culture—can impact decisions in purchasing supplies or tools that can impact patient safety, such as investing in more hemorrhage carts to improve access in the case of a hemorrhage event. The organization's values can also influence how the physical environment is designed in terms of light, layout and sound levels, which also influences the safety of patients and workers. Similarly, the design of technologies can change the likelihood of errors and harm [62], and the beliefs and values of an organization's culture are likely to influence what technology they purchase and implement. The external environment, for example, the rules and regulations related to Medicare and Medicaid reimbursement, may influence the values of the organization. As described in the SEIPS model, changes to one or more work system element impacts the others, which in turn changes how the care processes unfold.

Our finding coincides with the predictors of safety violations identified by Alper and Karsh, who performed a systematic review of safety violations across multiple industries [63]. In this review, Alper and Karsh defined safety violations as non-malevolent actions (i.e., actions that were not intended to harm or damage the system) [63]. The authors identified six categories of predictors of safety violations: individual characteristics, information or training, design to support worker needs, safety climate, competing goals, and problems with rules [39,64]. Table 3 maps examples of these predictors of safety violations to the work system elements. As shown in Table 3, the predictors of safety violations are related to the team, tasks, tools and technologies, and organization elements—with the organization element being the most common. We expect that the tools and technologies element was not proximally related to the emergent properties, but instead, it was distally related (i.e., it creates the potential for a work system barrier or facilitator but is not the immediate cause) [38]. This expectation is supported by the four facilitators in the Communication property, in which the participants mentioned that they use pagers to communicate that help is needed for an ongoing hemorrhage situation. While the physical and external environments were not highlighted in our findings, given that all elements of the work system shape processes and outcomes, our assumption is that these elements could be involved, and alternative methods (e.g., observation) might uncover the impact of the physical environment or the involvement of other stakeholders in other levels of the organizational leadership, but not involved in the direct provision of care, might identify the impact of rules and regulations outside the organization.

Table 3. Mapping between work system elements and predictors of safety violations.

Work System Element	Definition [33,35,37,39]	Predictors of Safety Violations [63]
Person/Team	• The individual or team (e.g., a group of individuals), at the center of the system	• Individual attitude toward compliance with safety practices
Tasks	• The tasks performed by the team. The tasks may vary by content and variety and may have varying characteristics (e.g., physical and psychological demands)	• Competing tasks or goals
Tools and Technologies	• The tools and technologies used to perform tasks. These tools and technologies can be simple, e.g., paper, or complex (e.g., electronic health record)	• Inadequate tools
Organization	• The formal and informal organization, organizational culture and climate, and the leadership and management	• Training related to safety practices • Staffing levels • Management attitude toward compliance with safety practices • Outdated rules or procedures
Physical Environment	• The physical layout or design (e.g., workstation design, noise, lighting, etc.)	• None
External Environment	• Extra-organizational factors that may influence policy, standards, or characteristics of the health care domain	• None

4.2. Strategies to Improve Safety Culture

Overall, our study participants identified more positive aspects than negative related to safety culture, perhaps suggesting that they experience a positive safety culture currently, which positively influences their actions and behaviors. However, the negative aspects indicate that safety culture, the process involved in postpartum hemorrhage care, and potentially patient outcomes could be improved by redesigning the work system to mitigate the barriers.

Work system redesign using the SEIPS model has been performed in many empirical studies spanning several health care settings. For example, the SEIPS model has been used to analyze existing work systems in nursing homes [65,66], care transitions [59,67–70], and inpatient hospitals [71]. The SEIPS model has also been used to identify work system design principles and interventions in nursing homes [72] and pharmacies [73,74]. Results of a work system analysis can then be used to design and develop interventions [75], ensuring fit with the rest of the work system to avoid disrupting workflow [76] and creating negative, unanticipated consequences [50]. In this study, social-based interventions seem to be highlighted—having adequate staff to respond to a hemorrhage, especially to allow one experienced clinician familiar with policies at this health care system, facilitated a swift, positive response to the hemorrhage and was indicative of a positive safety culture. So, hospital management might ensure that an experienced nurse—perhaps a charge nurse—is empowered to step away from charge duties, perhaps delegating to an individual of their choosing or someone already designated and helping to organize a hemorrhage response. Of course, delegating charge duties to another nurse would involve a handoff and lead to negative consequences on other work activities. From a technology perspective, a checklist shown on a shared, smart display, updated either automatically (based on sensors) or by a designated individual in the hemorrhage response, that shows the suggested workflow and role responsibilities during a hemorrhage response could support teamwork, communication, and awareness of suggested organizational processes. In developing and implementing these solutions, one could close the feedback loop, allowing safety culture to inform the design of the work system as well as the design of the work system shaping safety culture.

Outside of SEIPS-based analysis, other systems engineering techniques could be leveraged to facilitate hemorrhage response specifically or safety culture more generally [77]. For example, Lean Thinking could help to ensure the availability of resources (including staff) and thus improve safety culture. Lean Thinking, developed by the Toyota Motor Corporation as a strategy to optimize auto manufacturing in the United States, consists of concepts, methods, and tools to eliminate unnecessary waste and minimize delays in work [78,79]. Lean Thinking is commonly implemented in EDs to mitigate similar obstacles to those identified in our study (e.g., delays in providing care, difficulties in communication, and poor patient safety) [78–82]. Several empirical articles demonstrate significant improvements in patient outcomes after Lean Thinking Principles have been implemented. For example, in 2011, Holden performed a literature review of 18 empirical studies of EDs that implemented Lean Thinking. He found that implementing Lean Thinking in EDs led to various care process changes, such as staffing changes and new technologies and communication systems to support patient care [78]. A similar systematic literature review study was performed in 2021 by Souza and colleagues. They found that implementing Lean Thinking in EDs led to reductions in waiting time, patient flow, and procedure times, as well as improvements in efficiency, productivity, and patient safety [83]. Examples of Lean Principles that were implemented in the ED to mitigate barriers similar to the barriers identified by our participants include:

- Staffing Shortages: Division of medical and nursing staff to work on specific patient streams [78,84–86], altering staffing schedules to reassign physicians and nurses to match peak patient volume [78,87], and redefining responsibilities of medical and nursing staff [78,88].
- Communication and Teamwork: Implementing communication tools [78,87].

5. Conclusions

In this study, we explored how factors related to safety culture help and hinder the response to postpartum hemorrhage—a leading cause of maternal mortality in the United States and worldwide. Adequate staffing, adequate and efficient communication, organizational management and leadership, clear and salient organizational processes, and good teamwork were all related to positive safety culture in hemorrhage responses. Additional opportunities, targeting both social and technical subsystems of the sociotechnical system in postpartum hemorrhage response, could build upon these results. Ultimately, our study provides additional empirical evidence that the design of the sociotechnical system shapes safety culture—and closing feedback loops by designing, developing, and implementing sociotechnical-based solutions shows how safety culture can shape the sociotechnical system.

This study does indeed have some limitations. As highlighted in the discussion, triangulating multiple data streams (e.g., including observation) and/or interviewing additional stakeholders in the organization who do not directly provide care but do influence hemorrhage response processes might uncover additional emergent properties that influence safety culture. Further, including some review of actual patient outcomes via chart review and a survey-based measure of safety culture would have helped to gain a deeper understanding of the safety culture at this site. Importantly, we did not interview any patients, who would have important insights into safety culture and should be included in the future. Lastly, this study aimed to focus on postpartum hemorrhage at one participating health care site—our findings may not generalize to other sites, and a careful comparison of contexts is needed.

Author Contributions: Conceptualization, W.F.B. and A.R.W.; methodology, K.L.H.-L. and A.R.W.; software, K.L.H.-L.; validation, W.F.B., N.V. and S.C.; formal analysis, K.L.H.-L., M.M.S. and A.R.W.; investigation, K.L.H.-L. and R.E.-A.; resources, R.E.-A. and A.R.W.; data curation, K.L.H.-L.; writing—original draft preparation, K.L.H.-L. and A.R.W.; writing—review and editing, M.M.S., N.V., S.C., R.E.-A. and W.F.B.; visualization, K.L.H.-L., supervision, A.R.W. and W.F.B.; project administration, R.E.-A.; funding acquisition, A.R.W. and W.F.B. All authors have read and agreed to the published version of the manuscript.

Funding: This work was funded by the Jump ARCHES endowment through the Health Care Engineering Systems Center under grant number P363.

Institutional Review Board Statement: Ethical review and approval were waived for this study due to the Peoria IRB Board determining that it does not meet the definition of research under the purview of the IRB according to federal regulations on 3 May 2023.

Informed Consent Statement: Informed consent for participation is not required as per federal legislation as this study did not meet the definition of research, however verbal assent was obtained from all participants involved in the study.

Data Availability Statement: The data presented in this study are available on request from the corresponding author due to participant confidentiality concerns.

Acknowledgments: We thank our study participants, as our work would not be possible without them. We would also like to thank Adviye Irem Yuceel, who assisted with interview logistics, transcription, and cleaning and Jonathan Handler, who is involved in the larger study. We give thanks to the original caretakers of the land where we performed this study. The University of Illinois at Urbana-Champaign occupies the lands of the Peoria, Kaskaskia, Piankashaw, Wea, Miami, Mascoutin, Odawa, Sauk, Mesquaki, Kickapoo, Potawatomi, Ojibwe, and Chickasaw Nations.

Conflicts of Interest: All authors declare no conflicts of interest. The funders had no role in the design of the study; in the collection, analyses, or interpretation of data; in the writing of the manuscript; or in the decision to publish the results.

Abbreviations

The following abbreviations are used in this manuscript:

SEIPS	Systems Engineering Initiative for Patient Safety
STS	Sociotechnical system
OB/GYN	Obstetrics and gynecology
CST	Certified surgical technologists
PCT	Patient care technicians

References

1. Lagrew, D.; McNulty, J.; Sakowski, C.; Cape, V.; McCormick, E.; Morton, C. *Improving Health Care Response to Obstetric Hemorrhage, a California Maternal Quality Care Collaborative Toolkit*; CMQCC: Palo Alto, CA, USA, 2022.
2. Tikkanen, R.; Gunja, M.Z.; FitzGerald, M.; Zephyrin, L.C. Maternal Mortality and Maternity Care in the United States Compared to 10 Other Developed Countries. *Commonw. Fund* **2020**, *10*, 22. [CrossRef]
3. ACOG American College of Obstetricians and Gynecologists. Postpartum Hemorrhage (Practice Bullen No. 183) 2017. Available online: https://www.acog.org/clinical/clinical-guidance/practice-bulletin/articles/2017/10/postpartum-hemorrhage (accessed on 27 February 2024).
4. Andrikopoulou, M.; D'Alton, M.E. Postpartum hemorrhage: Early identification challenges. *Semin. Perinatol.* **2019**, *43*, 11–17. [CrossRef] [PubMed]
5. Ekin, A.; Gezer, C.; Solmaz, U.; Taner, C.E.; Dogan, A.; Ozeren, M. Predictors of severity in primary postpartum hemorrhage. *Arch. Gynecol. Obs.* **2015**, *292*, 1247–1254. [CrossRef] [PubMed]
6. Ende, H.B.; Butwick, A.J. Current State and Future Direction of Postpartum Hemorrhage Risk Assessment. *Obs. Gynecol.* **2021**, *138*, 924–930. [CrossRef] [PubMed]
7. Main, E.K.; McCain, C.L.; Morton, C.H.; Holtby, S.; Lawton, E.S. Pregnancy-related mortality in California: Causes, characteristics, and improvement opportunities. *Obstet. Gynecol.* **2015**, *125*, 938–947. [CrossRef] [PubMed]
8. Dahlke, J.D.; Mendez-Figueroa, H.; Maggio, L.; Hauspurg, A.K.; Sperling, J.D.; Chauhan, S.P.; Rouse, D.J. Prevention and management of postpartum hemorrhage: A comparison of 4 national guidelines. *Am. J. Obstet. Gynecol.* **2015**, *213*, 76.e1–76.e10. [CrossRef]
9. Vogel, J.P.; Nguyen, P.-Y.; Ramson, J.; De Silva, M.S.; Pham, M.D.; Sultana, S.; McDonald, S.; Adu-Bonsaffoh, K.; McDougall, A.R.A. Effectiveness of care bundles for prevention and treatment of postpartum hemorrhage: A systematic review. *Am. J. Obstet. Gynecol.* **2024**, *231*, 67–91. [CrossRef] [PubMed]
10. Main, E.K.; Cape, V.; Abreo, A.; Vasher, J.; Woods, A.; Carpenter, A.; Gould, J.B. Reduction of severe maternal morbidity from hemorrhage using a state perinatal quality collaborative. *Am. J. Obstet. Gynecol.* **2017**, *216*, 298.e1–298.e11. [CrossRef] [PubMed]
11. Gallos, I.; Devall, A.; Martin, J.; Middleton, L.; Beeson, L.; Galadanci, H.; Alwy Al-beity, F.; Qureshi, Z.; Hofmeyr, G.J.; Moran, N.; et al. Randomized Trial of Early Detection and Treatment of Postpartum Hemorrhage. *N. Engl. J. Med.* **2023**, *389*, 11–21. [CrossRef]
12. Henrich, W.; Dückelmann, A.; Braun, T.; Hinkson, L. Uterine packing with chitosan-covered tamponade to treat postpartum hemorrhage. *Am. J. Obs. Gynecol.* **2024**, *230*, S1061–S1065. [CrossRef] [PubMed]
13. Henriquez, D.D.C.A.; Bloemenkamp, K.W.M.; van der Bom, J.G. Management of postpartum hemorrhage: How to improve maternal outcomes? *J. Thromb. Haemost.* **2018**, *16*, 1523–1534. [CrossRef] [PubMed]
14. McLintock, C. Prevention and treatment of postpartum hemorrhage: Focus on hematological aspects of management. *Hematol. Am. Soc. Hematol. Educ. Program* **2020**, *2020*, 542–546. [CrossRef] [PubMed] [PubMed Central]
15. Collins, P.; Abdul-Kadir, R.; Thachil, J.; for The Subcommittees on Women' s Health Issues in Thrombosis and Haemostasis and on Disseminated Intravascular Coagulation. Management of coagulopathy associated with postpartum hemorrhage: Guidance from the SSC of the ISTH. *J. Thromb. Haemost. JTH* **2016**, *14*, 205–210. [CrossRef] [PubMed]
16. Schein, E.H. *Organizational Culture and Leadership*, 2nd ed.; Jossey-Bass: San Francisco, CA, USA, 1992.
17. Geertz, C. *The Interpretation of Cultures*; Basic Books: New York, NY, USA, 1973.
18. Carayon, P.; Xie, A. Decision making in healthcare system design: When human factors engineering meets health care. In *Cultural Factors in Decision Making and Action*; Proctor, R.W., Nof, S.Y., Yih, Y., Eds.; Taylor & Franci: Boca Raton, FL, USA, 2011; pp. 219–238.
19. Parker, S.K.; Van den Broeck, A.; Holman, D. Work Design Influences: A Synthesis of Multilevel Factors that Affect the Design of Jobs. *Acad. Manag. Ann.* **2016**, *11*, 267–308. [CrossRef]
20. Schneider, B.; Ehrhart, M.G.; Macey, W.H. Organizational Climate and Culture. *Annu. Rev. Psychol.* **2013**, *64*, 361–388. [CrossRef] [PubMed]
21. Guldenmund, F. Organizational safety culture. In *The Wiley Blackwell Handbook of the Psychology of Occupational Safety and Workplace Health*; Wiley Blackwel: Hoboken, NJ, USA, 2016; pp. 437–458.
22. AHRQ Agency for Healthcare Research and Quality. Hospital Survey on Patient Safety Culture Rockville, MD2023. Available online: https://www.ahrq.gov/sops/surveys/hospital/index.html (accessed on 5 June 2024).
23. Halligan, M.; Zecevic, A. Safety culture in healthcare: A review of concepts, dimensions, measures and progress. *BMJ Qual. Saf.* **2011**, *20*, 338–343. [CrossRef] [PubMed]
24. Bisbey, T.M.; Kilcullen, M.P.; Thomas, E.J.; Ottosen, M.J.; Tsao, K.; Salas, E. Safety Culture: An Integration of Existing Models and a Framework for Understanding Its Development. *Hum. Factors* **2021**, *63*, 88–110. [CrossRef] [PubMed]

25. World Health Organization. *Global Patient Safety Action Plan 2021–2030: Towards Eliminating Avoidable Harm in Health Care*; World Health Organization: Geneva, Switzerland, 2021.
26. Bishop, A.; Fleming, M.; Flin, R. Patient Safety Culture. In *The Wiley Blackwell Handbook of the Psychology of Occupational Safety and Workplace Health*; Wiley Blackwel: Hoboken, NJ, USA, 2015; pp. 459–484.
27. Carayon, P.; Hancock, P.; Leveson, N.; Noy, I.; Sznelwar, L.; van Hootegem, G. Advancing a sociotechnical systems approach to workplace safety—Developing the conceptual framework. *Ergonomics* **2015**, *58*, 548–564. [CrossRef] [PubMed]
28. Pronovost, P.; Ravitz, A.; Stoll, R.; Kennedy, S. Transforming Patient Safety: A Sector-Wide Systems Approach. Report of the WISH Patient Safety Forum. 2015. Available online: https://www.imperial.ac.uk/media/imperial-college/institute-of-global-health-innovation/public/Patient-safety.pdf (accessed on 23 December 2024).
29. International Ergonomics Association (IEA). The Discipline of Ergonomics 2000. Available online: https://iea.cc/about/what-is-ergonomics/ (accessed on 22 August 2004).
30. Mumford, E. The story of socio-technical design: Reflections on its successes, failures and potential. *Inf. Syst. J.* **2006**, *16*, 317–342. [CrossRef]
31. Kleiner, B.M. Macroergonomics: Analysis and design of work systems. *Appl. Ergon.* **2006**, *37*, 81–89. [CrossRef]
32. Hendrick, H.W.; Kleiner, B.M. *Macroergonomics—An Introduction to Work System Design*; The Human Factors and Ergonomics Society: Santa Monica, CA, USA, 2001.
33. Smith, M.J.; Carayon-Sainfort, P. A balance theory of job design for stress reduction. *Int. J. Ind. Ergon.* **1989**, *4*, 67–79. [CrossRef]
34. Carayon, P.; Smith, M.J. Work organization and ergonomics. *Appl. Ergon.* **2000**, *31*, 649–662. [CrossRef] [PubMed]
35. Carayon, P. The balance theory and the work system model... Twenty years later. *Int. J. Hum.–Comput. Interact.* **2009**, *25*, 313–327. [CrossRef]
36. Carayon, P.; Hundt, A.S.; Karsh, B.T.; Gurses, A.P.; Alvarado, C.J.; Smith, M.; Flatley Brennan, P. Work system design for patient safety: The SEIPS model. *Qual. Saf. Health Care* **2006**, *15*, i50–i58. [CrossRef] [PubMed]
37. Carayon, P.; Wooldridge, A.; Hoonakker, P.; Hundt, A.S.; Kelly, M.M. SEIPS 3.0: Human-centered design of the patient journey for patient safety. *Appl. Ergon.* **2020**, *84*, 103033. [CrossRef]
38. Holden, R.J.; Carayon, P.; Gurses, A.P.; Hoonakker, P.; Hundt, A.S.; Ozok, A.A.; Rivera-Rodriguez, A.J. SEIPS 2.0: A human factors framework for studying and improving the work of healthcare professionals and patients. *Ergonomics* **2013**, *56*, 1669–1686. [CrossRef] [PubMed] [PubMed Central]
39. Carayon, P.; Wetterneck, T.B.; Rivera-Rodriguez, A.J.; Hundt, A.S.; Hoonakker, P.; Holden, R.; Gurses, A.P. Human factors systems approach to healthcare quality and patient safety. *Appl. Ergon.* **2014**, *45*, 14–25. [CrossRef] [PubMed] [PubMed Central]
40. Wilson, J.R. Fundamentals of systems ergonomics/human factors. *Appl. Ergon.* **2014**, *45*, 5–13. [CrossRef]
41. Johnson, C.W. What are emergent properties and how do they affect the engineering of complex systems? *Reliab. Eng. Syst. Saf.* **2006**, *91*, 1475–1481. [CrossRef]
42. Dekker, S.W.A.; Hancock, P.A.; Wilkin, P. Ergonomics and sustainability: Towards an embrace of complexity and emergence. *Ergonomics* **2013**, *56*, 357–364. [CrossRef] [PubMed]
43. Werner, N.E.; Malkana, S.; Gurses, A.P.; Leff, B.; Arbaje, A.I. Toward a process-level view of distributed healthcare tasks: Medication management as a case study. *Appl. Ergon.* **2017**, *65*, 255–268. [CrossRef] [PubMed]
44. Carayon, P.; Gurses, A.P.; Hundt, A.S.; Ayoub, P.; Alvarado, C.J. Performance Obstacles Facilitators of Healthcare Providers. In *Change and Quality in Human Service Work*; Korunka, C., Hoffmann, P., Eds.; Hampp Publishers: Munchen, Germany, 2005; pp. 257–276.
45. Brown, K.A.; Mitchell, T.R. A comparison of just-in-time and batch manufacturing: The role of performance obstacles. *Acad. Manag. J.* **1991**, *34*, 906–917. [CrossRef]
46. Brown, K.A.; Mitchell, T.R. Performance obstacles for direct and indirect labour in high technology manufacturing. *Int. J. Prod. Res.* **1988**, *26*, 1819–1832. [CrossRef]
47. Peters, L.H.; O'Connor, E.J. Situational constraints and work outcomes: The influences of a frequently overlooked construct. *Acad. Manag. Rev.* **1980**, *5*, 391–397. [CrossRef]
48. Hettinger, L.J.; Kirlik, A.; Goh, Y.M.; Buckle, P. Modelling and simulation of complex sociotechnical systems: Envisioning and analysing work environments. *Ergonomics* **2015**, *58*, 600–614. [CrossRef] [PubMed] [PubMed Central]
49. Robertson, M.M.; Hettinger, L.J.; Waterson, P.E.; Noy, Y.I.; Dainoff, M.J.; Leveson, N.G.; Carayon, P.; Courtney, T.K. Sociotechnical approaches to workplace safety: Research needs and opportunities. *Ergonomics* **2015**, *58*, 650–658. [CrossRef] [PubMed]
50. Wooldridge, A.R.; Morgan, J.; Ramadhani, W.A.; Hanson, K.; Vazquez-Melendez, E.; Kendhari, H.; Shaikh, N.; Riech, T.; Mischler, M.; Krzyzaniak, S.; et al. Interactions in Sociotechnical Systems: Achieving Balance in the Use of an Augmented Reality Mobile Application. *Hum. Factors* **2024**, *66*, 658–682. [CrossRef]

51. Weiler, D.T.; Lingg, A.J.; Eagan, B.R.; Shaffer, D.W.; Werner, N.E. Quantifying the qualitative: Exploring epistemic network analysis as a method to study work system interactions. *Ergonomics* **2022**, *65*, 1434–1449. [CrossRef]
52. Salmon, P.M.; Walker, G.H.; MRead, G.J.; Goode, N.; Stanton, N.A. Fitting methods to paradigms: Are ergonomics methods fit for systems thinking? *Ergonomics* **2017**, *60*, 194–205. [CrossRef]
53. Hale-Lopez, K.L.; Saenz, M.M.; Verma, N.; Chakravarthy, S.; Handler, J.A.; Ebert-Allen, R.; Bond, W.F.; Wooldridge, A.R. A Macroergonomic Analysis to Identify Improvements to Postpartum Hemorrhage Anticipation, Identification, and Management. Under Review.
54. Robson, C.; McCartan, K. *Real World Research*, 4th ed.; Wiley & Sons Ltd.: West Sussex, UK, 2016.
55. Zoom. 2024. Available online: https://www.zoom.com/en (accessed on 17 February 2025).
56. Dedoose. 2024. Available online: https://www.dedoose.com/ (accessed on 17 February 2025).
57. Devers, K.J. How will we know "good" qualitative research when we see it? Beginning the dialogue in health services research. *Health Serv. Res.* **1999**, *34*, 1153–1188. [PubMed] [PubMed Central]
58. Creswell, J.W.; Creswell, J.D. *Research Design: Qualitative, Quantitative, and Mixed Methods Approaches*, 5th ed.; SAGE Publications: Los Angeles, CA, USA, 2018.
59. Wooldridge, A.R.; Carayon, P.; Hoonakker, P.; Hose, B.Z.; Eithun, B.; Brazelton, T., 3rd; Ross, J.; Kohler, J.E.; Kelly, M.M.; Dean, S.M.; et al. Work system barriers and facilitators in inpatient care transitions of pediatric trauma patients. *Appl. Ergon.* **2020**, *85*, 103059. [CrossRef] [PubMed] [PubMed Central]
60. Salas, E.; Cooke, N.; Rosen, M. On teams, teamwork, and team performance: Discoveries and developments. *Hum. Factors* **2008**, *50*, 540–547. [CrossRef]
61. Carayon, P.; Wust, K.; Hose, B.-Z.; Salwei, M.E. Human Factors and Ergonomics in Health care. In *Handbook of Human Factors and Ergonomics*, 5th ed.; Wiley & Sons: Hoboken, NJ, USA, 2021; pp. 1417–1437.
62. Carayon, P.; Wetterneck, T.B.; Schoofs-Hundt, A.; Ozkaynak, M.; DeSilvey, J.; Ludwig, B.; Ram, P.; Rough, S.S. Evaluation of nurse interaction with bar code medication administration technology in the work environment. *J. Patient Saf.* **2007**, *3*, 34–42. [CrossRef]
63. Alper, S.J.; Karsh, B.-T. A systematic review of safety violations in industry. *Accid. Anal. Prev.* **2009**, *41*, 739–754. [CrossRef]
64. Altabbakh, H.; AlKazimi, M.A.; Murray, S.; Grantham, K. STAMP—Holistic system safety approach or just another risk model? *J. Loss Prev. Process Ind.* **2014**, *32*, 109–119. [CrossRef]
65. Ford, J.H.; Jolles, S.A.; Heller, D.; Langenstroer, M.; Crnich, C. There and back again: The shape of telemedicine in U.S. nursing homes following COVID-19. *BMC Geriatr.* **2022**, *22*, 337. [CrossRef]
66. Powell, K.R.; Winkler, A.E.; Liu, J.; Alexander, G.L. A mixed-methods analysis of telehealth implementation in nursing homes amidst the COVID-19 pandemic. *J. Am. Geriatr. Soc.* **2022**, *70*, 3493–3502. [CrossRef]
67. Abraham, J.; Meng, A.; Sona, C.; Wildes, T.; Avidan, M.; Kannampallil, T. An observational study of postoperative handoff standardization failures. *Int. J. Med. Inform.* **2021**, *151*, 104458. [CrossRef]
68. Oh, S.; Sang, E.; Stawnychy, M.A.; Garren, P.; You, S.B.; O'Connor, M.; Hirschman, K.B.; Hodgson, N.; Cranston, T.; Jablonski, J. Application of a Human Factors and Systems Engineering Approach to Explore Care Transitions of Sepsis Survivors From Hospital to Home Health Care. *Hum. Factors* **2024**, *66*, 2468–2484. [CrossRef]
69. Werner, N.E.; Rutkowski, R.; Graske, A.; Finta, M.K.; Sellers, C.R.; Seshadri, S.; Shah, M.N. Exploring SEIPS 2.0 as a model for analyzing care transitions across work systems. *Appl. Ergon.* **2020**, *88*, 103141. [CrossRef] [PubMed]
70. Wooldridge, A.R.; Carayon, P.; Hoonakker, P.; Hose, B.Z.; Schroeer, K.; Brazelton, T.; Eithun, B.; Rusy, D.; Ross, J.; Kohler, J.; et al. Care transition of trauma patients: Processes with articulation work before and after handoff. *Appl. Ergon.* **2022**, *98*, 103606. [CrossRef] [PubMed]
71. Mulac, A.; Mathiesen, L.; Taxis, K.; Gerd Granås, A. Barcode medication administration technology use in hospital practice: A mixed-methods observational study of policy deviations. *BMJ Qual. Amp. Saf.* **2021**, *30*, 1021–1030. [CrossRef] [PubMed]
72. Strauven, G.; Vanhaecht, K.; Anrys, P.; De Lepeleire, J.; Spinewine, A.; Foulon, V. Development of a process-oriented quality improvement strategy for the medicines pathway in nursing homes using the SEIPS model. *Res. Soc. Adm. Pharm.* **2020**, *16*, 360–376. [CrossRef]
73. Musuuza, J.S.; Fong, E.; Lata, P.; Willenborg, K.; Knobloch, M.J.; Hoernke, M.J.; Spiel, A.R.; Tischendorf, J.S.; Suda, K.J.; Safdar, N. Feasibility of a pharmacy-led intervention to de-implement non-guideline-concordant proton pump inhibitor use. *Implement. Sci. Commun.* **2021**, *2*, 59. [CrossRef] [PubMed]
74. Odukoya, O.K.; Stone, J.A.; Chui, M.A. Barriers and facilitators to recovering from e-prescribing errors in community pharmacies. *J. Am. Pharm. Assoc.* **2015**, *55*, 52–58. [CrossRef]
75. Carayon, P.; Hose, B.-Z.; Wooldridge, A.; Brazelton, T.B.; Dean, S.M.; Eithun, B.L.; Kelly, M.M.; Kohler, J.E.; Ross, J.; Rusy, D.A.; et al. Human-centered design of team health IT for pediatric trauma care transitions. *Int. J. Med. Inform.* **2022**, *162*, 104727. [CrossRef]

76. Salwei, M.E.; Carayon, P. A Sociotechnical Systems Framework for the Application of Artificial Intelligence in Health Care Delivery. *J. Cogn. Eng. Decis. Mak.* **2022**, *16*, 194–206. [CrossRef] [PubMed]
77. Carayon, P.; Wooldridge, A.R.; Hose, B.-Z.; Salwei, M.; Benneyan, J. Challenges And Opportunities For Improving Patient Safety Through Human Factors And Systems Engineering. *Health Aff.* **2018**, *37*, 1862–1869. [CrossRef]
78. Holden, R.J. Lean thinking in emergency departments: A critical review. *Ann. Emerg. Med.* **2011**, *57*, 265–278. [CrossRef] [PubMed]
79. Austin, E.E.; Blakely, B.; Tufanaru, C.; Selwood, A.; Braithwaite, J.; Clay-Williams, R. Strategies to measure and improve emergency department performance: A scoping review. *Scand. J. Trauma Resusc. Emerg. Med.* **2020**, *28*, 55. [CrossRef] [PubMed] [PubMed Central]
80. Kellermann, A.L. Crisis in the emergency department. *N. Engl. J. Med.* **2006**, *355*, 1300. [CrossRef] [PubMed]
81. Smits, M.; Groenewegen, P.P.; Timmermans, D.R.; van der Wal, G.; Wagner, C. The nature and causes of unintended events reported at ten emergency departments. *BMC Emerg. Med.* **2009**, *9*, 16. [CrossRef]
82. System CotFoECitUSH. *Hospital-Based Emergency Care: At the Breaking Point*; National Academies Press: Washington, DC, USA, 2007.
83. Souza, D.L.; Korzenowski, A.L.; Alvarado, M.M.; Sperafico, J.H.; Ackermann, A.E.F.; Mareth, T.; Scavarda, A.J. A Systematic Review on Lean Applications' in Emergency Departments. *Healthcare* **2021**, *9*, 763. [CrossRef] [PubMed]
84. Kelly, A.-M.; Bryant, M.; Cox, L.; Jolley, D. Improving emergency department efficiency by patient streaming to outcomes-based teams. *Aust. Health Rev.* **2007**, *31*, 16–21. [CrossRef] [PubMed]
85. King, D.L.; Ben-Tovim, D.I.; Bassham, J. Redesigning emergency department patient flows: Application of lean thinking to health care. *Emerg. Med. Australas.* **2006**, *18*, 391–397. [CrossRef] [PubMed]
86. Woodward, G.; Godt, M.; Fisher, K. Children's hospital and regional medical center emergency department patient flow—Rapid process improvement (RPI). In *Improving Healthcare Quality Using Toyota Lean Production Methods*; ASQ Quality Press: Milwaukee, WI, USA, 2007; Volume 46, pp. 145–150.
87. Eller, A. Rapid assessment and disposition: Applying LEAN in the emergency department. *J. Healthc. Qual. (JHQ)* **2009**, *31*, 17–22. [CrossRef]
88. Dickson, E.W.; Singh, S.; Cheung, D.S.; Wyatt, C.C.; Nugent, A.S. Application of lean manufacturing techniques in the emergency department. *J. Emerg. Med.* **2009**, *37*, 177–182. [CrossRef] [PubMed]

healthcare

MDPI

Opinion

Sailing Too Close to the Wind? How Harnessing Patient Voice Can Identify Drift towards Boundaries of Acceptable Performance

Siri Wiig [1,*], Catherine Jane Calderwood [2] and Jane O'Hara [3]

1 SHARE—Centre for Resilience in Healthcare, Faculty of Health Sciences, N-4036 Stavanger, Norway
2 Faculty of Science, University of Strathclyde, Glasgow G1 1XQ, UK; ccalderwood@doctors.org.uk
3 The Healthcare Improvement Studies (THIS) Institute, University of Cambridge, Cambridge CB1 8RN, UK; jane.o'hara@thisinstitute.cam.ac.uk
* Correspondence: siri.wiig@uis.no

Abstract: This opinion paper investigates how healthcare organizations identify and act upon different types of risk signals. These signals may generally be acknowledged, but we also often see with hindsight that they might not be because they have become a part of normal practice. Here, we detail how risk signals from patients and families should be acknowledged as system-level safety critical information and as a way of understanding and changing safety culture in healthcare. We discuss how healthcare organizations could work more proactively with patient experience data in identifying risks and improving system safety.

Keywords: deviance; drift; safety boundaries; patient voice

1. Introduction

Healthcare organizations unknowingly accept the increased risk of adverse events resulting from the cumulative effect of small reductions in care quality [1]. When signals are not identified and acted upon, organizations can drift towards the safety margins due to the normalization of deviance, including unacceptable staff and leadership behavior and performance [2,3]. As well as signaling problems in their own care, the experiences of patients and families can also be conceived as early warning signals of poor performance at the wider system level, either as negative single cases, or as general patterns of poor performance in the organizations. Here, we detail how these signals should be acknowledged as system-level safety critical information and as a way of understanding and changing safety culture in healthcare. We discuss how healthcare organizations could work more proactively with patient experience data in identifying risks and improving system safety. If they do not, they are most likely to encounter an organizational drift where the risk is uncontrolled.

2. Normalization of Deviance and Organizational Drift—What Is It?

In the safety science literature, there are numerous cases showing how signals of unsafe performance and deviance from safe work practices were identified, escalated, ignored, and eventually normalized over time. For example, staff may report near misses, unreliable work practices, inadequate staffing, failing technical equipment, or omitted safety procedures. Over time, particularly if these issues do not lead to adverse events, the suboptimal work practice continues, and the deviance becomes normal practice within the work culture. Whilst these small incremental erosions in the standards of practice might not be regarded in and of themselves as threatening safety, the many small omissions and adaptations leading to suboptimal practice can sometimes result in disaster. Outside of healthcare, this has been seen in high-profile events such as the Challenger explosion [3], the Deepwater horizon blowout [4], and other well-documented tragic safety events (e.g., Chernobyl, Costa Concordia).

A seemingly universal truth is that in the aftermath of such major accidents, early warning signals of the likelihood of catastrophic failure are identified. Early warning signals can be conceived as small signs of system performance or properties (e.g., technical, procedural, cultural, hierarchical) that may indicate or contribute to future failure. What is evident in the aftermath of such accidents is that these signals had been ignored or overlooked and came to be accepted as an unproblematic part of everyday work. In safety science terms, this could be conceived as the systematic erosion of the safety margins, leading to the drift towards a state where safety failures are more likely. Put simply, they had operated too close to the boundaries of acceptable performance, and this was culturally accepted as part of everyday work. Without a continued systematic assessment of performance, organizations, and individuals, they cannot know when they are too close to these boundaries before it is too late [2]. In this paper, we argue that patients' and families' voices represent an untapped resource to support the closer monitoring of organizations' proximity to the acceptable boundary of performance.

3. Adverse Outcomes in Healthcare Resulting from Organizational Drift

Within England, there have been several inquiries arising from concerns of systematic poor care and outcomes in maternity services. These inquiries consistently demonstrate similar failures happening repeatedly, despite warnings from families and staff [5–7]. Other examples from healthcare are also highly relevant in understanding the normalization of deviance and drift into failure [8]. For example, several 'whistleblowers' had raised concerns about the Bristol cardiac pediatric surgery unit prior to its investigation in 2001, but no action was taken in response. Subsequent investigations uncovered evidence of significant organizational and cultural problems in the healthcare environment, with punitive management styles, surgeons who lacked professional insight but continued working, and data not matching their view were discarded thus resulting in 30–35 children dying between 1991 and 1995 [9]. The Mid Staffordshire and Morecambe Bay inquiries showed similar patterns and recommendations focusing on the need for organizational and cultural changes [7,10]. These examples collectively illustrate how healthcare organizations (or at least parts of organizations) were operating within a degraded mode for years due to then normalization of unacceptable behaviors and performance, and with work cultures having limited interest in monitoring signals from staff, and patients and families, indicating that something was terribly wrong.

Understanding where an organization is operating in relation to acceptable performance boundaries is not straightforward [11] and requires information not just about 'breaches' of the boundary (safety incidents, formal patient complaints), but also identification of risk as well as constant enquiry. That enquiry should extend to the smaller, repeated failures that are often highlighted by the patient experience of care—failure to be treated with dignity and respect, of receiving basic levels of care—as well as the patient-reported harm events, which are formally reported to and handled by the organizations themselves, as well as a range of regulatory bodies in different healthcare systems. These repeated failures were evident within all the reports from the major inquiries, alongside parallel missed opportunities to learn and intervene that could have reduced the significant harm that resulted [7,9,10]. For example, families who gave birth at Morecambe Bay were often told that theirs was an isolated case, or that investigations had shown there was nothing that could have been carried out. There was evidence of uncaring practices, with staff showing little regard for those using their services. Sadly, many similar issues have been discovered elsewhere. Both Morecambe Bay and the Mid Staffordshire inquiries demonstrate how small, repeated failures were not considered as indicative of or relating to safety. We contend therefore that these 'early warning signals'—poor quality care, lack of dignity and respect—might collectively have indicated the drift into unacceptable performance, which in turn lays the foundations for these organizational disasters [7,10]. Both inquiry reports provide a real sense that if these 'early warning signals' were taken seriously, and as an indication of drift, the serious safety failings might not have happened. This also means that many of the deaths could have been prevented if signals from patients and families (individual and aggregated) were valued and acted upon by professionals and leaders. This needs to change as we see the same trends being repeated today, decades later [6].

4. Discussion

Safety critical industries have long acknowledged the need to identify, address, and use these types of early warning signals in a systemic approach to improve safety. Thinking about the road ahead, we contend that healthcare needs to recognize that it too is a safety critical industry and act in a more proactive way on signals from those who receive care. To understand how safe a healthcare organization is, we argue that the safety concerns and care experience of patients' and family's data goes beyond 'soft intelligence' [12] and should instead be conceived as fundamental safety critical information. In this final section, we outline the ways in which healthcare might move towards a systematic gathering and acting upon this safety critical intelligence from patient and families.

First, healthcare needs to systematize and legitimize information from patients and families as credible safety information to support their safety and care at the individual and system levels. Examples of these types of approaches include 'safety netting' and 'red flag' initiatives to manage diagnostic uncertainty in primary care [13]. Within acute care settings, a recent high-profile example within the UK is the implementation of 'Martha's Rule'. Martha Mills died of sepsis in 2021, aged 13, following a pancreatic injury sustained from the handlebar when she fell off her bike. Her family repeatedly expressed concern regarding her deteriorating condition and, in 2023, a coroner ruled that Martha would probably have survived if she had been moved to intensive care earlier. This new initiative aims to support both families and staff to access a rapid critical care review should they have concerns regarding the condition of a patient. It also promotes the systematic gathering of information from patients and families about their condition at least daily, using methods such as the 'patient wellness questionnaire' [14]. Such initiatives start to bridge the gap between individual signals of safety, which have been recognized as important for some time, and the wider system signals by integrating this as 'business as usual' alongside the more traditional methods of assessment, especially of a deteriorating patient (e.g., early warning systems).

Second, healthcare needs to use the available data from patients and families more systematically. Patient complaints are an established process within healthcare systems globally but are often seen as individual cases rather than a source of early warning signals. However, there is some evidence of the application of a validated, standardized approach to using patient complaints to identify 'hot spots' and 'blind spots' for patient harm within the Irish healthcare system [15]. Such approaches reconceptualize complaints as potential early warning signals.

Third, healthcare needs to systematically gather, attend to, and act on the plethora of data provided by patients and their families about the quality and safety of care outside of formal complaint systems. This was termed over a decade ago as the 'patient experience cloud' [16] to describe the large and ever-expanding source of data that are shared every day via the internet—and especially on social media—from people describing their experience of the quality and safety of healthcare. Importantly, there is emergent evidence that this cloud of data is associated with, and potentially predictive of, objective measures of quality including readmission rates, mortality, and infection rates [16,17]. The potential sources of these data on patient experience are enormous, and go beyond social media, extending to sites that systematically invite and curate patient and family experiences of health and social care. An example of this is Care Opinion, which is a free to access, non-profit website operating in an increasing number of health systems globally. It invites patients and families to leave feedback (anonymously if preferred) about their experience of health and social care. Using this platform, a recent study demonstrated that an automated analysis of the language used provides an outlet for reporting safety issues that may have been unnoticed or unresolved within formal channels [18]. The advances in automation of free text analysis [19] provide a potential mechanism for the systematic use of such sources by service providers, policymakers, and regulators to identify and potentially prevent organizational drift in healthcare.

Finally, to harness these concerns and experiences routinely to avoid operational failure will require resources, infrastructure, and design, as well accepting these sources of data as credible safety critical information. It is useful here to think about epistemic injustice [20]—whose voices are credible, sought out, and valued? Some studies have begun to explore this in relation to investigatory and regulatory processes following patient harm [17,21], where patients' and families' perspectives have been shown to differ from the healthcare professionals' and are often devalued compared to the views of the 'more competent' actors. Epistemic injustice is likely therefore to be an important consideration when advocating for better monitoring and proactive use of patients' experiences and information to prevent the breach of safety boundaries. Levers to support this systematization might include policy development and implementation, but also regulation [17]. The regulatory logic needs to move from an occupation with 'objective' evidence to the assessment of 'soft' signals [22]. This means a combination of regulatory measures to mandate the use of these types of information sources as part of work practices among the regulated organizations, as well as regulators who are interested and use this information to a stronger degree themselves as sources when monitoring system and organizational performance [17,23]. We acknowledge that this is difficult, but we believe that a careful and thoughtful approach as indicated above is needed and should be codesigned to better use these untapped sources of information.

5. Conclusions

Listening to and acting on the experiences of patients and families at both the individual and system levels may help reduce hierarchy and the risk of services crossing the boundary of acceptable performance; of 'sailing too close to the wind'. As Don Berwick stated in his 2013 report on improving the safety of patients within the NHS—"*Hear the patient voice, at every level, even when that voice is a whisper.*" [24] (p. 17). However, achieving this systematically will require resources, new healthcare and regulatory infrastructure, and work culture changes.

6. Future Directions

The future direction in this field requires a culture where healthcare organizations work more proactively with patient experience data in identifying risks, preventing the normalization of deviance, and improving system safety using all available sources.

Author Contributions: Author S.W. had the idea together with J.O. and C.J.C. S.W. drafted the first version of the manuscript, followed by significant input and contributions from C.J.C. and J.O. All authors have read and agreed to the published version of the manuscript.

Funding: J.O. is supported by funding from the National Institute for Health and Care Research (NIHR) Yorkshire and Humber Patient Safety Research Collaboration (PSRC). The views expressed are those of the author(s) and not necessarily those of the NIHR or the Department of Health and Social Care.

Institutional Review Board Statement: Not applicable.

Informed Consent Statement: Not applicable.

Data Availability Statement: No new data were created or analyzed in this study.

Conflicts of Interest: The authors declare no conflicts of interest.

References

1. Vincent, C.; Amalberti, R. *Progress and Challenges for Patient Safety. In Safer Healthcare*; Springer: Cham, Switzerland, 2016; pp. 1–12.
2. Rasmussen, J. Risk management in a dynamic society: A modelling problem. *Saf. Sci.* **1997**, *27*, 183–213. [CrossRef]
3. Vaughan, D. *The Challenger Launch Decision: Risky Technology, Culture, and Deviance at NASA*; University of Chicago Press: Chicago, IL, USA, 1996.
4. CSB. *Investigation Report Executive Summary. Drilling Rig Explosion and Fire at the Macondo Well*; U.S. Chemical Safety and Hazard Investigation Board: Washington, DC, USA, 2016.
5. Dixon-Woods, M.; Barry, Z.; McGowan, J.; Martin, G. The state of care in England's maternity services. *BMJ* **2023**, *283*, 2700. [CrossRef] [PubMed]
6. Ockenden, D. *Ockenden Report Final. Final Findings, Conclusions and Essential Actions from the Ockenden Review of Maternity Services at Shrewsbury and Telford Hospital NHS Trust*; Department of Health & Social Care: London, UK, 2022.
7. Kirkup, B. *The Report of the Morecambe BAY Investigation*; The Stationery Office: London, UK, 2015.
8. Dekker, S. *Drift into Failure*; Routledge: Boca Raton, FL, USA, 2011.
9. Kennedy, I. *The Report of the Public Inquiry into Children's Heart Surgery at the Bristol Royal Infirmary 1984–1995 Learning from Bristol*; Bristol Royal Infirmary Inquiry: Bristol, UK, 2001.
10. Francis, R. *Report of the Mid Staffordshire NHS Foundation Trust Public Inquiry Volume 1: Analysis of evidence and lessons learned (Part 1)*; The Stationery Office: London, UK, 2013.
11. Cook, R.; Rasmussen, J. "Going solid": A model of system dynamics and consequences for patient safety. *BMJ Qual. Saf.* **2005**, *142*, 130–134. [CrossRef] [PubMed]
12. Martin, G.P.; McKee, L.; Dixon-Woods, M. Beyond metrics? Utilizing 'soft intelligence' for healthcare quality and safety. *Soc. Sci. Med.* **2015**, *142*, 19–26. [CrossRef] [PubMed]
13. Greenhalgh, S.; Finucane, L.M.; Mercer, C.; Selfe, J. Safety netting; best practice in the face of uncertainty. *Musculoskelet. Sci. Pract.* **2020**, *48*, 102179. [CrossRef] [PubMed]
14. Albutt, A.; O'Hara, J.; Conner, M.; Lawton, R. Can Routinely Collected, Patient-Reported Wellness Predict National Early Warning Scores? A Multilevel Modeling Approach. *J. Patient Saf.* **2021**, *17*, 548–552. [CrossRef] [PubMed]
15. O'Dowd, E.; Lydon, S.; Lambe, K.; Vellinga, A.; Rudland, C.; Ahern, E.; Hilton, A.; Ward, M.E.; Kane, M.; Reader, T.; et al. An analysis of complaints about hospital care in the Republic of Ireland. *Int. J. Qual. Health Care* **2022**, *34*, mzac037. [CrossRef] [PubMed]
16. Greaves, F.; Pape, U.J.; King, D.; Darzi, A.; Majeed, A.; Wachter, R.M.; Millett, C. Associations between Web-Based Patient Ratings and Objective Measures of Hospital Quality. *Arch. Intern. Med.* **2012**, *172*, 435–436. [CrossRef] [PubMed]
17. Wiig, S.; Rutz, S.; Boyd, A.; Churruca, K.; Kleefstra, S.; Haraldseid-Driftland, C.; Braithwaite, J.; O'Hara, J.; van de Bovenkamp, H. What methods are used to promote patient and family involvement in healthcare regulation? A multiple case study across four countries. *BMC Health Serv. Res.* **2020**, *20*, 616. [CrossRef] [PubMed]
18. Gillespie, A.; Reader, T. Online patient feedback as a safety valve: An automated language analysis of unnoticed and unresolved safety incidents. *Risk Anal.* **2023**, *43*, 1463–1477. [CrossRef] [PubMed]
19. Khanbhai, M.; Anyadi, P.; Symons, J.; Flott, K.; Darzi, A.; Mayer, E. Applying natural language processing and machine learning techniques to patient experience feedback: A systematic review. *BMJ Health Care Inform.* **2021**, *28*, e100262. [CrossRef] [PubMed]
20. Fricker, M. *Epistemic Injustice. Power and the Ethics of Knowing*; Oxford University Press: Oxford, UK, 2009.
21. Kok, J.H.; Leistikow, I.P.; Bal, R. Patient and family engagement in incident investigations: Exploring hospital manager and incident investigators' experiences and challenges. *J. Health Serv. Res. Policy* **2018**, *23*, 252–261. [CrossRef] [PubMed]
22. Wiig, S.; Aase, K.; Bal, R. Reflexive spaces: Leveraging resilience into healthcare regulation and management. *J. Patient Saf.* **2021**, *17*, e1681–e1684. [CrossRef] [PubMed]
23. Kok, J.; Wallenburg, I.; Leistikov, I.; Bal, R. The doctor was rude, the toilets are dirty. Utilizing 'soft signals' in the regulation of patient safety. *Saf. Sci.* **2020**, *131*, 104914. [CrossRef]
24. Berwick, D. *A Promise to Learn—A Commitment to Act. Improving the Safety of Patients in England*; National Advisory Group on the Safety of Patients in England: London, UK, 2013.

healthcare

MDPI

Article

Speaking Up and Taking Action: Psychological Safety and Joint Problem-Solving Orientation in Safety Improvement

Hassina Bahadurzada [1,*], Michaela Kerrissey [2] and Amy C. Edmondson [1]

[1] Harvard Business School, Harvard University, Soldiers Field Road, Boston, MA 02162, USA
[2] Harvard TH Chan School of Public Health, Harvard University, 677 Huntington Ave, Boston, MA 02115, USA
* Correspondence: hbahadurzada@hbs.edu

Abstract: Healthcare organizations face stubborn challenges in ensuring patient safety and mitigating clinician turnover. This paper aims to advance theory and research on patient safety by elucidating how the role of psychological safety in patient safety can be enhanced with joint problem-solving orientation (JPS). We hypothesized and tested for an interaction between JPS and psychological safety in relation to safety improvement, leveraging longitudinal survey data from a sample of 14,943 patient-facing healthcare workers. We found a moderation effect, in which psychological safety was positively associated with safety improvement, and the relationship was stronger in the presence of JPS. Psychological safety and JPS also interacted positively in predicting clinicians' intent to stay with the organization. For theory and research, our findings point to JPS as a measurable factor that may enhance the value of psychological safety for patient safety improvement—perhaps because voiced concerns about patient safety often require joint problem-solving to produce meaningful change. For practice, our conceptual framework, viewing psychological safety and JPS as complementary factors, can help organizations adopt a more granular approach towards assessing the interpersonal aspect of their safety climate. This will enable organizations to obtain a more nuanced understanding of their safety climate and identify areas for improvement accordingly.

Keywords: patient safety; psychological safety; joint problem-solving orientation; clinician turnover; safety climate

1. Introduction

Amid considerable progress, improving safety remains a priority in healthcare. Safety events resulting in serious, and sometimes fatal, outcomes are common [1]. Recent estimates in the US indicate that one in four adverse events is preventable [2]. These findings underscore the need to better understand the factors that enable improvements in safety and how to best foster safety in practice.

The frequency and substantial impact of medical errors over many years have inspired work on safety climate in healthcare [3,4]. Safety climate is defined as staff perceptions and attitudes reflecting the priority placed on safety in an organization [5,6]. Safety climate is regarded as key to delivering safe care because perceptions and attitudes about safety shape clinician and staff behaviors in the process of care delivery at a given point in time [5]. Safety climate is considered the surface feature of an underlying safety culture, which comprises the staff's shared values about the importance of safety, their beliefs about how things operate in their organization, and behavioral norms prioritizing safety [7,8].

Safety climate has effectively been measured in healthcare and has been associated with fewer errors and better patient and clinician outcomes [9–11]. This climate is characterized by senior management's commitment to safety, the use of resources to address safety, the clarity of norms regarding patient safety standards, and interpersonal dynamics among clinicians and staff [5,6]. Healthcare organizations with safety climates are seen to prioritize safety and learning by encouraging frontline staff to adhere to protocols, seek clarification when needed, share insights, report errors and near misses, and engage in learning to enhance safety. Although prior research has explored multiple aspects of safety climates, we lack understanding of how psychological safety and other interpersonal factors lead to material improvements in patient safety.

1.1. Background: Psychological Safety and the Surfacing of Safety Concerns

A vital interpersonal aspect of a safety climate is psychological safety—a state of low interpersonal risk that helps people feel able to ask questions, request help, and admit mistakes [12]. Psychological safety has been widely studied in teams across a variety of settings and is associated with beneficial outcomes, such as improved information sharing [13,14], enhanced willingness to voice concerns [15], and enhanced team learning [12,16–18]. Psychological safety matters for safety climate because it helps frontline staff voice safety concerns and encourages learning from incidents [19,20]. When people are afraid to speak up about errors, incidents, and near misses, these issues often go undetected, undermining a team's ability to learn from them and improve safety in the future. In addition to these learning-oriented benefits, frontline staff who perceive their environment as psychologically safe report enhanced wellbeing [21] and reduced emotional exhaustion [22].

Psychological safety is especially needed in the context of healthcare delivery because professional hierarchy and functional diversity, both features of healthcare work, create substantial barriers to speaking up [23,24]. Many good ideas voiced by staff with the intention to improve work processes do not reach fruition because they are rejected by managers and senior leaders without consideration [25]. Other good ideas are embraced initially but become lost in the complex hierarchical structures that characterize most large, multi-layered health systems [26]. Research has found that psychological safety can mitigate the barriers imposed by hierarchy [23], functional diversity [27], and professional boundaries [28]. By reducing the perceived interpersonal risk for raising questions and ideas, psychological safety can help people more easily speak up across professional hierarchies and functional diversity.

1.2. Research Gap: From Surfacing Safety Concerns to Addressing Safety Concerns through Joint Problem-Solving

While frontline staff voicing safety concerns and reporting errors matter for improving patient safety, voice alone does not ensure that safety concerns will be addressed [29]. The complexity of healthcare often means that problems leading to safety events and near misses have multiple causes and involve more than one person [30]. Addressing voiced concerns or errors effectively may require diverse functional and technical experts to team up and determine what to do. Recent organizational scholarship points to a need to better understand what occurs after the moment of voice in organizations, especially with team membership fluidity [26]. In fluid and dynamic work settings, collaborative problem-solving can be hard to generate, because individual clinicians and staff work through shifting schedules and rotating patient panels throughout their days [31]. Even well-intentioned individuals willing to raise a concern, admit a mistake, or ask a question may find themselves frustrated and stymied by what happens next if they feel unable to spur changes that might enhance safety.

Recent research on joint problem-solving orientations in fluid teams offers Joint problem-solving orientation (JPS) as one potential factor that may help realize the benefits of psychological safety for patient safety improvement. Joint problem-solving orientation is defined as emphasizing problems as shared and viewing solutions as requiring co-production [32]. Research in hospitals has found that JPS varies significantly across units and that those with higher JPS exhibit greater perceived care quality and safety [33]. The positive relationship between JPS and quality and safety is partially mediated through recognition and appreciation of one another's skills and knowledge, facilitating the quick surfacing and integration of task-relevant knowledge. This preliminary work developing the concept of JPS in healthcare suggests that it may be relevant to improving safety and complementary to the established role of psychological safety.

1.3. New Contribution and Significance of the Study

In this paper we proceed in two steps. First, we expand the existing base of literature on the interpersonal aspect of a safety climate by presenting a conceptual model of psychological safety and joint problem-solving orientation and proposing how, individually and together, they promote safety improvement and worker retention in healthcare. Second, we conduct an exploratory test of these relationships using empirical data from a large healthcare organization in the US.

2. Conceptual Model and Hypotheses

We conceptualize psychological safety and joint problem-solving orientation as complementary interpersonal factors that contribute to *patient safety improvement* and frontline staff's *intent to stay* with an organization. Figure 1 depicts our conceptualization of psychological safety and JPS as complementary by placing each on an axis from low to high, indicating how both can co-occur to a high degree (the upper right-hand quadrant) or a low degree (the lower left-hand quadrant). We suggest, in addition, that individuals may have a mix, represented on the off-diagonal, whereby individuals perceive high psychological safety with little JPS or the converse. These two features may be important to consider together in improving safety because they are each related to improvement behavior and engagement and may interact in ways that further support patient safety.

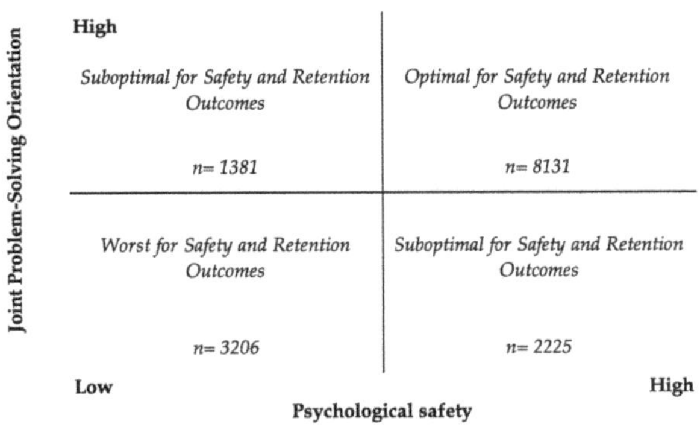

Note: respondents who agreed or strongly agreed on the presence of psychological safety and JPS were categorized as high.

Figure 1. Psychological safety and joint problem-solving orientation.

We proceeded with three main hypotheses based on this model (Figure 2). The first pertains to replicating previous findings associating psychological safety with patient safety [34–36], particularly expanding the link to safety *improvement*. To define safety improvement, we drew on process-change literature, which notes that change requires active intervention and choice [37,38]. We view safety improvement as a type of process change in healthcare, one that is defined by active intervention with the aim of improving safety. To make safety improvement, employees must perceive the environment as safe for speaking up. Frontline staff's input is increasingly valued in quality and safety improvement efforts because they may notice issues that would be otherwise missed [39–41]. To offer this input, frontline clinicians and staff must be willing to speak up about what they see [42]. Psychological safety—a state of low interpersonal risk—means frontline staff can speak up without fear of reprisal [12]. Healthcare organizations where frontline staff feel comfortable speaking up demonstrate higher quality decision-making and quicker error detection [43], enhanced quality improvements and safety [44], and increased employee motivation and commitment to the organization [19]. Therefore, we hypothesized that a safe interpersonal climate in which speaking up is expected and encouraged is associated with greater safety improvement and higher intent to stay.

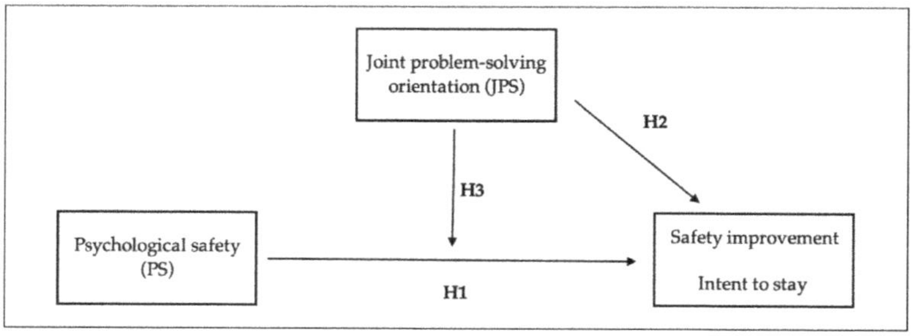

Figure 2. Hypothesized research model.

H1: *Psychological safety is associated with a greater level of safety improvement (H1a) and intent to stay (H1b).*

Our second hypothesis considers the role of joint problem-solving (JPS) in safety improvement. Team membership fluidity in healthcare has been shown to pose challenges to team performance, including safety performance, in part because voicing safety concerns is unlikely to be sufficient to make safety improvements when action is required [26]. Coordinated action to make changes is difficult when team member fluidity is high and differences across functions and expertise lead to the potential for disconnect [45]. JPS describes the perception that challenges are shared, along with a willingness to resolve them together [32,33,46].

Healthcare delivery takes place in a highly specialized environment where timely access to required skills and expertise matters, as does adherence to rules and procedures in pursuit of achieving safe and high-quality care [47,48]. The interdependence of the work, which requires multiple areas of expertise, puts a premium on rapidly establishing awareness of what other expertise domains can contribute. JPS may enhance care safety and quality by helping staff and clinicians understand their interdependence and value the diversity of expertise that others bring [33]. For example, recognizing the value that others offer may lead to more input-seeking behavior, facilitating collaboration in resolving safety concerns and thereby increasing the likelihood of effective safety improvement. We hypothesized that JPS creates a supportive environment, leading to a higher clinician intent to stay and more safety improvement, as the collective crafting of solutions is more likely to reach implementation and enhance safety.

H2: *Joint problem-solving orientation is associated with a greater level of safety improvement (H2a) and intent to stay (H2b).*

We further posited a positive interaction from the presence of both psychological safety and JPS. When frontline staff speak up and raise concerns and see addressing them as a collective responsibility, this is likely to improve patient care and spur employee engagement in improvement initiatives [32]. Speaking up without support from colleagues for solving problems together may nonetheless occur, stemming from a range of factors, such as professional communication barriers, complex organization structures, power dynamics, or a lack of resources. If these issues are not appropriately addressed, frontline staff may feel ignored or disrespected, prompting them to choose silence in the future [49,50]. Work settings where people feel a degree of JPS but are nonetheless afraid to speak up are also problematic for safety improvement—in these settings, people may expect to collaborate but feel unable to admit errors or report near misses, thus focusing instead on improvement that is less interpersonally risky. We hypothesized that when frontline staff perceive a collective responsibility for addressing safety concerns in their work environment, voiced safety concerns are more likely to be addressed and clinicians will display a higher commitment to the organization.

H3: *A joint problem-solving orientation positively moderates how psychological safety relates to safety improvement (H3a) and clinician intent to stay (H3b).*

3. Methods

3.1. Setting and Sample

The data for this research were obtained from a large multi-site health system with their main location in the United States. The health system administers a bi-annual electronic census survey to all employees in English to examine their perception of their work environment. Our data were collected in 2019 (n = 42,196, response rate = 87%) and 2021 (n = 50,471, response rate = 80%). We only retained respondents for whom we had data on our measures at both time points and excluded all individuals in purely administrative roles, so as to focus on frontline staff (n = 14,943). This exclusion was made because frontline staff's exposure to direct patient care makes their perception of safety especially important for patient safety outcomes [5]. Respondents in our analytical sample identified primarily as physicians, nurses, advanced practice clinicians, or allied health professionals.

3.2. Measurement Variables

3.2.1. Independent Variable

Psychological safety was measured using four survey items reflecting the extent to which respondents felt safe to speak up when confronted with issues within their organization, as measured in 2019. The items were adapted from the psychological safety scale originally used by Edmondson (1999) [12], with modifications to reflect a particular context of healthcare delivery in which patient safety and patient care are central. The items included (1) "I can report patient safety mistakes without fear of punishment", (2) "I feel free to raise workplace safety concerns", (3) "Caregivers will freely speak up if they see something that may negatively affect patient care", and (4) "Caregivers feel free to question the decisions or actions of those with more authority". To obtain a comprehensive understanding of the perceived climate, the first two items were measured at the individual level and the latter two items at the organizational level. We calculated Cronbach's alpha (a = 0.79) to assess the internal consistency of the items. We computed the composite measure of psychological safety as a mean of these four variables.

3.2.2. Independent and Moderating Variable

Joint problem-solving orientation was adapted from a previously validated measure [32]. Through iterative input with organizational staff, the items measuring joint problem-solving orientation were modified from the original measure in order to reflect the healthcare delivery environment within the organization. It included three items assessing the extent to which employees perceived care delivery to be a collective effort with shared responsibility: (1) "We view addressing problems as a team effort in this department", (2) "When a problem arises, we routinely involve whomever is needed to address it, regardless of their unit or role", and (3) "We can rely on people in other departments to address problems with us when needed" (a = 0.86). All items used for this measure were captured in 2019.

3.2.3. Dependent Variables

Safety improvement examined the extent to which employees believed that safety improvement had been/was being made within their organization, as measured at two time points (2019 and 2021). We operationalized safety improvement as a composite measure of the following two items (calculated as a mean): (1) "In this organization, we are actively doing things to improve patient safety" and (2) "Mistakes have led to positive changes in this organization" (May 2019 $a = 0.82$; May 2021 $a = 0.84$). In line with past work on process change in healthcare [38], we focused on items that emphasized active change toward safety improvement in the organization.

Intent to stay was measured by assessing employees' commitment to remain with the organization. Frontline staff were asked to answer the item "I would stay with this organization if offered a similar position elsewhere" on a five-point Likert scale, ranging from strongly disagree (1) to strongly agree (5).

3.2.4. Control Variables

We obtained and controlled for the following respondent-level characteristics: sex, role, tenure, and race. Sex (0 = male; 1 = female) and race (0 = non-white; 1 = white) were included as binary variables. The respondent's role and tenure were included as categorical variables with reference categories of physician and tenure of less than one year, respectively.

3.3. Statistical Analysis

To create a longitudinal dataset tracking individuals, we merged the frontline staff survey data from 2019 and 2021 at the individual level. We performed descriptive analyses, examining univariate and bivariate statistics for each measure ($n = 14{,}943$). We calculated Cronbach's alpha for the composite measures of psychological safety, joint problem-solving orientation, and safety improvement to assess the internal consistency of the items pertaining to each construct. We computed correlations between the independent and dependent variables (Table 1). Joint problem-solving orientation exhibited a correlation of 0.67 with psychological safety, which is consistent with the complementary and reciprocal nature of the constructs.

Table 1. Sample characteristics ($n = 14{,}943$).

Characteristics	*n* (%)
Female	11,589 (77.55%)
Role	
Physician	2214 (14.82%)
Nurse	8024 (53.70%)
Advanced practice clinician	1019 (6.82%)
Allied health professional	3686 (24.67%)
Race	
White (not of Hispanic origin)	12,217 (81.76%)
Black or African American	1142 (7.64%)
Asian	810 (5.42%)
Hispanic or Latino	519 (3.47%)
Other	255 (1.71%)
Tenure	
Less than 1 year	1461 (9.78%)
Tenure 1–10 years	7929 (53.06%)
Tenure 11–20 years	3490 (23.36%)
Tenure >20 years	2063 (13.81%)

To examine our hypotheses, we conducted regression analyses, both cross-sectionally in 2019 to examine immediate relationships and longitudinally from 2019 to 2021 to examine the extent to which psychological safety was associated with the moderator and outcomes over time. For the cross-sectional models, all variables were derived from the 2019 survey data; for the longitudinal models, dependent variables were pulled from the 2021 survey data. To test our hypotheses, we ran baseline and interaction regression models at the individual level, clustering the standard errors at the team/department level to adjust for department-level variations (specified as distinct departments in unique locations, e.g., the Emergency Department in Hospital X). We used ordinary least squares (OLS) linear regression models to ease the interpretation of the models; hierarchical linear models yielded broadly consistent results (one moderation finding became slightly more significant; we thus view the OLS results as conservative). Control variables for gender, role, race, and tenure were included based on prior literature associating demographic and status characteristics with psychological safety [23,51,52]. All analyses were conducted using STATA version 18.

4. Results

The respondent characteristics of our sample are reported in Table 1. The majority of respondents identified as female (77.55%), and slightly over half reported being a nurse (53.70%). Most had a tenure of between 1 and 10 years (53.06%), with 9.78% reporting a tenure of less than one year and 37.17% a tenure of 11 years or more. Respondents mainly identified as white (81.76%), followed by 7.64% Black or African American, 5.42% Asian, and 3.47% Hispanic or Latino.

Table 2 presents the measure correlations, and Figure 3 presents the unadjusted association between psychological safety and JPS. The scatterplot illustrates how psychological safety and JPS are positively correlated and yet also commonly exhibit observations on the off-diagonal, i.e., with a respondent reporting high on one and low on the other.

Table 2. Correlations between independent and dependent measures.

	Psychological Safety (2019)	Joint Problem-Solving (2019)	Safety Improvement (2019)	Safety Improvement (2021)	Intent to Stay (2019)	Intent to Stay (2021)
Psychological safety (2019)	1	0.67 *	0.66 *	0.37 *	0.50 *	0.31 *
Joint problem-solving (2019)		1	0.52 *	0.33 *	0.49 *	0.30 *
Safety improvement (2019)			1	0.43 *	0.46 *	0.31 *
Safety improvement (2021)				1	0.29 *	0.49 *
Intent to stay (2019)					1	0.44 *
Intent to stay (2021)						1

Note: * corresponds to p-value < 0.01.

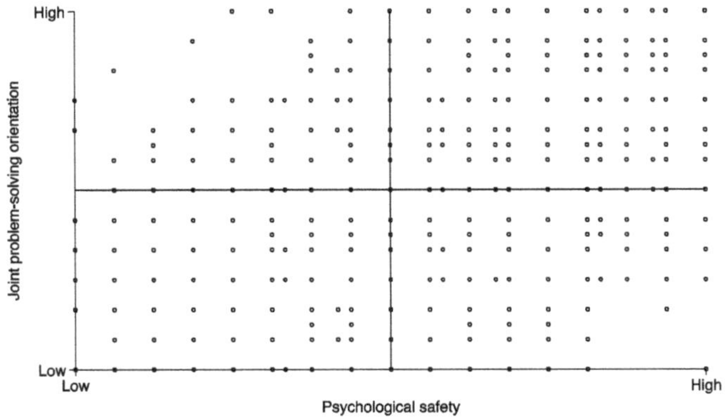

Figure 3. The relationship between psychological safety and JPS.

Table 3 presents the descriptive statistics for the measures of interest in this study. On average, respondents agreed to experiencing psychological safety (mean = 4.12, SD = 0.71). The mean for JPS was somewhat lower (mean = 3.92, SD = 0.82), on average qualitatively corresponding to not agreeing that they perceived a JPS orientation in their work unit. For the outcome measures, frontline staff perceived more safety improvement in 2019 (mean = 4.31, SD = 0.72) compared to 2021 (mean = 4.21, SD = 0.79), and a similar pattern was present for intent to stay (mean = 4.05, SD=0.97 in 2019; mean = 3.94, SD = 0.85 in 2021).

Table 3. Measure descriptions: *n*, mean, standard deviation (SD), and response distribution.

Measures	*n*	Mean	SD	Response Distribution (%)				
				1	2	3	4	5
Psychological safety (2019)	14,936	4.12	0.71					
Report patient safety mistakes without fear of punishment	14,671	4.37	0.85	1.45	2.91	6.94	34.94	53.77
Feel free to raise workplace safety concerns	14,886	4.32	0.82	1.07	2.81	7.78	40.20	48.15
Caregivers speak up if something negatively affects patient care	14,759	4.29	0.85	1.16	3.69	8.02	39.64	47.49
Caregivers feel free to question those with more authority	14,752	3.53	1.09	4.77	13.72	23.67	39.19	18.65
Joint problem-solving orientation (2019)	14,606	3.92	0.82					
View addressing problems as a team effort	14,547	3.94	0.96	1.97	7.34	15.40	45.25	30.05
Involve whomever needed to address the problem	14,416	3.99	0.91	1.65	5.69	14.73	47.96	29.97
Rely on people in other department to address problems with us	14,157	3.83	0.90	1.53	6.56	21.83	47.51	22.58
Safety improvement (2019)	14,855	4.31	0.72					
We are actively doing things to improve patient safety	14,818	4.38	0.77	0.88	1.88	7.22	38.39	51.63
Mistakes have led to positive changes	14,586	4.24	0.79	0.73	1.89	12.42	42.80	42.17
Safety improvement (2021)	14,865	4.21	0.79					
We are actively doing things to improve patient safety	14,834	4.27	0.86	1.51	2.96	9.30	39.31	46.93
Mistakes have led to positive changes	14,620	4.15	0.85	1.07	2.81	14.63	42.59	38.90
Intent to stay (2019)	14,790	4.05	0.90	1.16	3.56	20.22	39.67	35.38
Intent to stay (2021)	14,763	3.94	0.97	2.08	5.03	22.62	36.97	33.30

Table 4 displays the regression results, demonstrating consistent findings across both the cross-sectional and longitudinal models for the baseline and moderation analyses. Psychological safety and joint problem-solving orientation were consistently and statistically significantly associated with safety improvement and intent to stay ($p < 0.01$), in support of Hypotheses 1a and 1b, and 2a and 2b. The presence of higher levels of psychological safety and JPS were both associated with greater safety improvement and intent to stay. Using the cross-sectional models as an example, these relationships can be interpreted as follows: holding other variables constant, a one-point increase in psychological safety was associated with a 0.57-point increase in safety improvement and a 0.39-point increase in intent to stay; a one-point increase in JPS was associated with a 0.13-point increase in safety improvement and a 0.31-point increase in intent to stay.

Table 4. Models relating psychological safety (PS) and joint problem-solving (JPS) to safety improvement and intent to stay.

	Safety Improvement				Intent to Stay			
	Cross-Sectional		Longitudinal		Cross-Sectional		Longitudinal	
	Main Effect	Interaction	Main Effect	Interaction	Main Effect	Interaction	Main Effect	Interaction
Psychological safety (PS)	0.565 ***	0.485 ***	0.286 ***	0.186 ***	0.392 ***	0.049	0.276 ***	0.046
Joint problem-solving (JPS)	0.131 ***	0.040	0.162 ***	0.048	0.305 ***	−0.086 *	0.199 ***	−0.062
PS # JPS		0.023 **		0.028 ***		0.097 ***		0.065 ***
Female	0.018	0.020 *	0.023	0.025	0.028 *	0.035 **	0.026	0.030
Role								
Advanced practice provider	−0.040	−0.039 *	−0.148 ***	−0.146 ***	0.086 ***	0.092 ***	−0.054	−0.050
Nurse	−0.082 ***	−0.030 ***	−0.242 ***	−0.240 ***	0.143 ***	0.150 ***	−0.049 *	−0.044
Allied health professional	−0.083 ***	−0.082***	−0.185 ***	−0.184 ***	0.171 ***	0.177 ***	−0.029	−0.025
Tenure								
1–10 years	−0.007	−0.008	0.127 ***	0.126 ***	−0.075 ***	−0.079 ***	0.149 ***	0.147 ***
11–20 years	0.025	0.023	0.223 ***	0.221 ***	−0.030	−0.038	0.306 ***	0.301 ***
>20 years	0.073 ***	0.071 ***	0.278 ***	0.275 ***	0.060 **	0.052 **	0.439 ***	0.434 ***
White	0.011	0.012	−0.029	−0.028	−0.039 **	−0.035 **	0.035 *	0.038 *
Intercept	1.498 ***	1.807 ***	2.432 ***	2.820 ***	1.156 ***	2.485 ***	1.800 ***	2.690 ***
Number of observations	14,549	14,549	14,545	14,545	14,474	14,474	14,438	14,438
R-squared	0.45	0.45	0.17	0.17	0.30	0.31	0.13	0.13

Note: * corresponds to p-value < 0.10, ** corresponds to p-value < 0.05, and *** corresponds to p-value < 0.01.

We also found support for hypotheses 3a and 3b regarding the presence of moderation. The interaction models indicated that psychological safety had a positive significant relationship with safety improvement and that this relationship was stronger in the presence of JPS in both the cross-sectional ($\beta = 0.023$, $p < 0.01$) and longitudinal models ($\beta = 0.028$, $p < 0.01$). Keeping psychological safety constant, more safety improvement was experienced when respondents took collective responsibility for problems and co-produced solutions. For intent to stay, the moderation analyses demonstrated that the significant main effects of psychological safety and JPS on intent to stay became non-significant in the presence of their interaction. The significant interaction term, indicating a mutually reinforcing relationship between psychological safety and JPS on clinician intent to stay, was observed in both the cross-sectional ($\beta = 0.097$, $p < 0.01$) and longitudinal analyses ($\beta = 0.065$, $p < 0.01$).

5. Discussion and Conclusions

This study sought to understand how psychological safety and joint problem-solving orientation together help alleviate the stubborn challenges that healthcare systems face in seeking to ensure patient safety and reduce clinician turnover. Our analyses show that both psychological safety and JPS relate directly to enhanced safety improvement and clinician commitment to an organization, and we found evidence of moderation, whereby the effect of psychological safety was stronger in the presence of a joint problem-solving orientation. These findings advance our understanding of the interpersonal dynamics for the frontline workers who play a crucial role in influencing safety improvement, both through raising issues and by addressing them effectively together.

In prior research, psychological safety and JPS were shown to predict improvement behavior and engagement, but in this study, we propose a new theory to explain why they may interact in ways that further enhance patient safety. To examine the interaction between psychological safety and JPS, we conceptualized psychological safety and JPS as complementary by placing each on an axis from low to high, indicating how both can co-occur to a high degree (the upper right-hand quadrant) or a low degree (the lower left-hand quadrant). Additionally, individuals may experience a mix, which is represented on the off-diagonal, whereby they experience high psychological safety with little JPS, or the converse. Our findings support that the combined effect of psychological safety and JPS is greater than the sum of their individual effects. When psychological safety and JPS co-occur to a high degree (upper right-hand quadrant), frontline staff are committed to their organization and report greater safety improvement. We posit that the combined presence of JPS and psychological safety is especially effective for safety improvement because it enables issues to be raised *and* addressed together when needed. This builds on past research findings that JPS has both a direct relationship to safety and a relationship that is mediated through enhancing recognition of the value that other expertise areas offer [33]. When healthcare workers feel they can take interpersonal risks to raise issues and then solve them together, they are both better able to concretely address issues, and in the process, they may learn more about one another and how to work to improve and assure day-to-day safety.

There were some notable insights from our findings regarding the off-diagonals. In the quadrant with high psychological safety but low JPS, frontline staff may speak up without receiving input and support from colleagues for addressing the issues that are raised. For safety improvement, our findings suggest that beliefs about speaking up relate positively to patient safety, even independently of this joint support from colleagues (as indicated by the persistent main effect of psychological safety in the moderation model). This is plausible because not all safety concerns require collaborative efforts to be resolved—some are simple issues and/or can be independently addressed. In many healthcare organizations, voiced concerns posing an immediate or critical safety hazard prompt collective action through well-established processes, which are carefully developed and assiduously followed. In these certain instances where the threat is simple and/or quickly addressable, psychological safety is more likely to be sufficient to enhance safety.

In contrast, this persistent relationship between psychological safety and the outcome in the moderation model was not present when considering clinician intent to stay as the outcome. Other research has found that when frontline staff continue to speak up and raise concerns without response, input, and support from colleagues, they can feel ignored or disrespected, decreasing their engagement and exacerbating burnout [32,49]. Our data further emphasize the interdependence between psychological safety and JPS and show a mutually reinforcing relationship between both constructs. Psychological safety and JPS are interrelated in their relationship with clinicians' commitment to the organization. This was indicated by the statistically significant relationship for the interaction term between JPS and psychological safety and intent to stay.

Studies in other high-pressure environments have shown that improvement efforts tend to be centralized and hierarchical rather than collective and democratic [53–55]. This can be an efficient approach to improvement, drawing on the benefits of hierarchical coordination in organizations. However, our measure of psychological safety also points to risks in this approach—specifically, across the items comprising psychological safety, we noted that only half of the respondents reported feeling comfortable to question decisions and actions of those with more authority, a proportion markedly lower than the other items in the psychological safety measure. This indicates that attention to psychological safety in hierarchical safety reporting environments may be especially vital [56].

Our study offers theoretical and practical implications by emphasizing the importance of the interpersonal aspect of safety climates. We introduce JPS as a complementary factor to psychological safety when examining interpersonal dynamics in healthcare. With the introduction of JPS, we urge scholars to adopt a more nuanced approach in understanding how attitudes and cognitions are raised and addressed when needed. This approach can also help managers in healthcare, who can effectively monitor not only frontline staff's willingness to voice concerns but also their readiness to collaborate in tackling safety challenges together. Tailored solutions and interventions, thus, can be designed and implemented based on whether frontline staff are hesitant to express safety concerns or perceive a lack of collaborative efforts to address reported safety challenges. Therefore, our model provides opportunities to diagnose and improve a team or department.

This study has limitations. First, while we examined how psychological safety and JPS relate to one another and to patient and clinician outcomes, our models indicate associations and not causations. Furthermore, we found some evidence of a dynamic relationship between psychological safety and JPS but did not have access to sufficiently fine-grained longitudinal data to explore it directly. For safety improvement, the interaction coefficient increased over the two-year lag between our cross-sectional and longitudinal models, suggesting that high psychological safety and high JPS mutually reinforce one another over time. Future longitudinal studies can examine the feedback loop between psychological safety and JPS. Second, despite a large analytical sample across different geographic locations, our study was conducted within one large healthcare delivery organization with a shared mission and vision, which may limit the generalizability of our findings across other organizations. Third, we studied the relationship between psychological safety and JPS, but there are likely various other factors, such as hierarchy, human resource management systems, and safety policies, that may interact with psychological safety and JPS. Future research can examine how psychological safety and JPS together interact with other procedural and interpersonal factors to affect patient and clinician outcomes.

Our study emphasizes the importance of the interpersonal aspects of a safety climate in enhancing patient and clinician outcomes in healthcare. Interpersonal dynamics are important in all sectors, but in healthcare—a highly specialized sector—where effective collaboration and timely access to required skills and expertise save lives, interpersonal dynamics are vital to the quality and safety of care delivery.

Author Contributions: Formal analysis, H.B.; writing—original draft, H.B.; writing—review and editing, M.K. and A.C.E. All authors have read and agreed to the published version of the manuscript.

Funding: This research received no external funding.

Institutional Review Board Statement: Ethical review and approval were waived for this study. The study was classified as Not Human Subjects Research.

Informed Consent Statement: Not applicable to this study.

Data Availability Statement: The data for this study were made accessible to the authors by the organization through a data use agreement. The data are not publicly available. Requests for further information about the data can be directed to mkerrissey@hsph.harvard.edu.

Conflicts of Interest: The authors declare no conflict of interest.

References

1. Camargo, C.A.; Tsai, C.-L.; Sullivan, A.F.; Cleary, P.D.; Gordon, J.A.; Guadagnoli, E.; Kaushal, R.; Magid, D.J.; Rao, S.R.; Blumenthal, D. Safety Climate and Medical Errors in 62 US Emergency Departments. *Ann. Emerg. Med.* **2012**, *60*, 555–563.e20. [CrossRef] [PubMed]
2. Bates, D.W.; Levine, D.M.; Salmasian, H.; Syrowatka, A.; Shahian, D.M.; Lipsitz, S.; Zebrowski, J.P.; Myers, L.C.; Logan, M.S.; Roy, C.G.; et al. The Safety of Inpatient Health Care. *N. Engl. J. Med.* **2023**, *388*, 142–153. [CrossRef] [PubMed]
3. Committee on Quality of Healthcare in America. *Crossing the Quality Chasm: A New Health System for the 21st Century*; National Academies Press: Washington, DC, USA, 2001.
4. Havens, D.H.; Boroughs, L. "To Err Is Human": A Report from the Institute of Medicine. *J. Pediatr. Health Care* **2000**, *14*, 77–80.
5. Singer, S.; Lin, S.; Falwell, A.; Gaba, D.; Baker, L. Relationship of Safety Climate and Safety Performance in Hospitals. *Health Serv. Res.* **2009**, *44*, 399–421. [CrossRef]
6. Zohar, D. Safety Climate in Industrial Organizations: Theoretical and Applied Implications. *J. Appl. Psychol.* **1980**, *65*, 96–102. [CrossRef]
7. Flin, R. Measuring Safety Climate in Health Care. *Qual. Saf. Health Care* **2006**, *15*, 109–115. [CrossRef]
8. Naveh, E.; Katz-Navon, T.; Stern, Z. Treatment Errors in Healthcare: A Safety Climate Approach. *Manag. Sci.* **2005**, *51*, 948–960. [CrossRef]
9. Brewer, B.B. Relationships Among Teams, Culture, Safety, and Cost Outcomes. *West. J. Nurs. Res.* **2006**, *28*, 641–653. [CrossRef]
10. Clarke, S. The Relationship between Safety Climate and Safety Performance: A Meta-Analytic Review. *J. Occup. Health Psychol.* **2006**, *11*, 315–327. [CrossRef]
11. Stone, P.W.; Gershon, R.R.M. Nurse Work Environments and Occupational Safety in Intensive Care Units. *JONA J. Nurs. Adm.* **2009**, *39*, S27. [CrossRef]
12. Edmondson, A. Psychological Safety and Learning Behavior in Work Teams. *Adm. Sci. Q.* **1999**, *44*, 350–383. [CrossRef]
13. Collins, C.J.; Smith, K.G. Knowledge Exchange and Combination: The Role of Human Resource Practices in the Performance of High-Technology Firms. *Acad. Manag. J.* **2006**, *49*, 544–560. [CrossRef]
14. Siemsen, E.; Roth, A.V.; Balasubramanian, S.; Anand, G. The Influence of Psychological Safety and Confidence in Knowledge on Employee Knowledge Sharing. *Manuf. Serv. Oper. Manag.* **2009**, *11*, 429–447. [CrossRef]
15. Ashford, S.J.; Rothbard, N.P.; Piderit, S.K.; Dutton, J.E. Out on a Limb: The Role of Context and Impression Management in Selling Gender-Equity Issues. *Adm. Sci. Q.* **1998**, *43*, 23. [CrossRef]
16. Bunderson, J.S.; Boumgarden, P. Structure and Learning in Self-Managed Teams: Why "Bureaucratic" Teams Can Be Better Learners. *Organ. Sci.* **2010**, *21*, 609–624. [CrossRef]
17. Carmeli, A. Social Capital, Psychological Safety and Learning Behaviours from Failure in Organisations. *Long Range Plan.* **2007**, *40*, 30–44. [CrossRef]
18. Carmeli, A.; Gittell, J.H. High-quality Relationships, Psychological Safety, and Learning from Failures in Work Organizations. *J. Organ. Behav.* **2009**, *30*, 709–729. [CrossRef]
19. Edmondson, A.C.; Bransby, D.P. Psychological Safety Comes of Age: Observed Themes in an Established Literature. *Annu. Rev. Organ. Psychol. Organ. Behav.* **2023**, *10*, 55–78. [CrossRef]
20. Rosenbaum, L. Cursed by Knowledge—Building a Culture of Psychological Safety. *N. Engl. J. Med.* **2019**, *380*, 786–790. [CrossRef]
21. Kark, R.; Carmeli, A. Alive and Creating: The Mediating Role of Vitality and Aliveness in the Relationship between Psychological Safety and Creative Work Involvement. *J. Organ. Behav. Int. J. Ind. Occup. Organ. Psychol. Behav.* **2009**, *30*, 785–804. [CrossRef]
22. Rathert, C.; Ishqaidef, G.; Porter, T.H. Caring Work Environments and Clinician Emotional Exhaustion: Empirical Test of an Exploratory Model. *Health Care Manag. Rev.* **2022**, *47*, 58–65. [CrossRef] [PubMed]
23. Nembhard, I.M.; Edmondson, A.C. Making It Safe: The Effects of Leader Inclusiveness and Professional Status on Psychological Safety and Improvement Efforts in Health Care Teams. *J. Organ. Behav. Int. J. Ind. Occup. Organ. Psychol. Behav.* **2006**, *27*, 941–966. [CrossRef]

24. Detert, J.R.; Treviño, L.K. Speaking Up to Higher-Ups: How Supervisors and Skip-Level Leaders Influence Employee Voice. *Organ. Sci.* **2010**, *21*, 249–270. [CrossRef]
25. Fast, N.J.; Burris, E.R.; Bartel, C.A. Managing to Stay in the Dark: Managerial Self-Efficacy, Ego Defensiveness, and the Aversion to Employee Voice. *Acad. Manag. J.* **2014**, *57*, 1013–1034. [CrossRef]
26. Satterstrom, P.; Vogus, T.J.; Jung, O.S.; Kerrissey, M. Voice Is Not Enough: A Multilevel Model of How Frontline Voice Can Reach Implementation. *Health Care Manag. Rev.* **2024**, *49*, 35. [CrossRef] [PubMed]
27. Malhotra, M.K.; Ahire, S.; Shang, G. Mitigating the Impact of Functional Dominance in Cross-Functional Process Improvement Teams. *Decis. Sci.* **2017**, *48*, 39–70. [CrossRef]
28. Martins, L.L.; Schilpzand, M.C.; Kirkman, B.L.; Ivanaj, S.; Ivanaj, V. A Contingency View of the Effects of Cognitive Diversity on Team Performance: The Moderating Roles of Team Psychological Safety and Relationship Conflict. *Small Group Res.* **2013**, *44*, 96–126. [CrossRef]
29. Detert, J.R.; Burris, E.R.; Harrison, D.A.; Martin, S.R. Voice Flows to and around Leaders: Understanding When Units Are Helped or Hurt by Employee Voice. *Adm. Sci. Q.* **2013**, *58*, 624–668. [CrossRef]
30. Edmondson, A.C. Learning from Mistakes Is Easier Said Than Done: Group and Organizational Influences on the Detection and Correction of Human Error. *J. Appl. Behav. Sci.* **1996**, *32*, 5–28. [CrossRef]
31. Valentine, M.A.; Edmondson, A.C. Team Scaffolds: How Mesolevel Structures Enable Role-Based Coordination in Temporary Groups. *Organ. Sci.* **2015**, *26*, 405–422. [CrossRef]
32. Kerrissey, M.J.; Mayo, A.T.; Edmondson, A.C. Joint Problem-Solving Orientation in Fluid Cross-Boundary Teams. *Acad. Manag. Discov.* **2021**, *7*, 381–405. [CrossRef]
33. Kerrissey, M.J.; Novikov, Z. Joint Problem-Solving Orientation, Mutual Value Recognition, and Performance in Fluid Teamwork Environments. *Front. Psychol.* **2024**, *15*, 1288904. [CrossRef] [PubMed]
34. Belyansky, I.; Martin, T.R.; Prabhu, A.S.; Tsirline, V.B.; Howley, L.D.; Phillips, R.; Sindram, D.; Heniford, B.T.; Stefanidis, D. Poor Resident-Attending Intraoperative Communication May Compromise Patient Safety. *J. Surg. Res.* **2011**, *171*, 386–394. [CrossRef] [PubMed]
35. Leroy, H.; Dierynck, B.; Anseel, F.; Simons, T.; Halbesleben, J.R.B.; McCaughey, D.; Savage, G.T.; Sels, L. Behavioral Integrity for Safety, Priority of Safety, Psychological Safety, and Patient Safety: A Team-Level Study. *J. Appl. Psychol.* **2012**, *97*, 1273–1281. [CrossRef] [PubMed]
36. Rathert, C.; Ishqaidef, G.; May, D.R. Improving Work Environments in Health Care: Test of a Theoretical Framework. *Health Care Manag. Rev.* **2009**, *34*, 334. [CrossRef] [PubMed]
37. Carrillo, J.E.; Gaimon, C. Improving Manufacturing Performance Through Process Change and Knowledge Creation. *Manag. Sci.* **2000**, *46*, 265–288. [CrossRef]
38. Tucker, A.L.; Nembhard, I.M.; Edmondson, A.C. Implementing New Practices: An Empirical Study of Organizational Learning in Hospital Intensive Care Units. *Manag. Sci.* **2007**. [CrossRef]
39. Jung, O.S.; Kundu, P.; Edmondson, A.C.; Hegde, J.; Agazaryan, N.; Steinberg, M.; Raldow, A. Resilience vs. Vulnerability: Psychological Safety and Reporting of near Misses with Varying Proximity to Harm in Radiation Oncology. *Jt. Comm. J. Qual. Patient Saf.* **2021**, *47*, 15–22. [CrossRef]
40. Tucker, A.L.; Singer, S.J.; Hayes, J.E.; Falwell, A. Front-Line Staff Perspectives on Opportunities for Improving the Safety and Efficiency of Hospital Work Systems. *Health Serv. Res.* **2008**, *43*, 1807–1829. [CrossRef]
41. Morrison, E.W. Employee Voice and Silence. *Annu. Rev. Organ. Psychol. Organ. Behav.* **2014**, *1*, 173–197. [CrossRef]
42. Morrison, E.W. Employee Voice Behavior: Integration and Directions for Future Research. *Acad. Manag. Ann.* **2011**, *5*, 373–412. [CrossRef]
43. Morrison, E.W.; Milliken, F.J. Organizational Silence: A Barrier to Change and Development in a Pluralistic World. *Acad. Manag. Rev.* **2000**, *25*, 706–725. [CrossRef]
44. Robbins, J.; McAlearney, A.S. Toward a High-Performance Management System in Health Care, Part 5: How High-Performance Work Practices Facilitate Speaking up in Health Care Organizations. *Health Care Manag. Rev.* **2020**, *45*, 278. [CrossRef] [PubMed]
45. Salas, E.; Reyes, D.L.; McDaniel, S.H. The Science of Teamwork: Progress, Reflections, and the Road Ahead. *Am. Psychol.* **2018**, *73*, 593–600. [CrossRef] [PubMed]
46. Swinth, R.L. Organizational Joint Problem-Solving. *Manag. Sci.* **1971**, *18*, B68–B79. [CrossRef]
47. Hollnagel, E. *Safer Complex Industrial Environments: A Human Factors Approach*; CRC Press: Boca Raton, FL, USA, 2009.
48. Schaefer, H.G.; Helmreich, R.L.; Scheidegger, D. Human Factors and Safety in Emergency Medicine. *Resuscitation* **1994**, *28*, 221–225. [CrossRef] [PubMed]
49. Lainidi, O.; Jendeby, M.K.; Montgomery, A.; Mouratidis, C.; Paitaridou, K.; Cook, C.; Johnson, J.; Karakasidou, E. An Integrative Systematic Review of Employee Silence and Voice in Healthcare: What Are We Really Measuring? *Front. Psychiatry* **2023**, *14*, 1111579. [CrossRef] [PubMed]
50. Morrow, K.J.; Gustavson, A.M.; Jones, J. Speaking up Behaviours (Safety Voices) of Healthcare Workers: A Metasynthesis of Qualitative Research Studies. *Int. J. Nurs. Stud.* **2016**, *64*, 42–51. [CrossRef] [PubMed]
51. Garcia, L.C.; Shanafelt, T.D.; West, C.P.; Sinsky, C.A.; Trockel, M.T.; Nedelec, L.; Maldonado, Y.A.; Tutty, M.; Dyrbye, L.N.; Fassiotto, M. Burnout, Depression, Career Satisfaction, and Work-Life Integration by Physician Race/Ethnicity. *JAMA Netw. Open* **2020**, *3*, e2012762. [CrossRef]

52. McPeek-Hinz, E.; Boazak, M.; Sexton, J.B.; Adair, K.C.; West, V.; Goldstein, B.A.; Alphin, R.S.; Idris, S.; Hammond, W.E.; Hwang, S.E.; et al. Clinician Burnout Associated with Sex, Clinician Type, Work Culture, and Use of Electronic Health Records. *JAMA Netw. Open* **2021**, *4*, e215686. [CrossRef]
53. Driskell, J.E.; Salas, E. Group Decision Making under Stress. *J. Appl. Psychol.* **1991**, *76*, 473. [CrossRef]
54. Foushee, H.C.; Helmreich, R.L. 7—Group Interaction and Flight Crew Performance. In *Human Factors in Aviation*; Wiener, E.L., Nagel, D.C., Eds.; Cognition and Perception; Academic Press: San Diego, CA, USA, 1988; pp. 189–227, ISBN 978-0-08-057090-7.
55. Hermann, C.F. Some Consequences of Crisis Which Limit the Viability of Organizations. *Adm. Sci. Q.* **1963**, *8*, 61–82. [CrossRef]
56. Detert, J.R.; Burris, E.R. Leadership Behavior and Employee Voice: Is the Door Really Open? *Acad. Manag. J.* **2007**, *50*, 869–884. [CrossRef]

healthcare

MDPI

Viewpoint

Why Talking Is Not Cheap: Adverse Events and Informal Communication

Anthony Montgomery [1,*], Olga Lainidi [2] and Katerina Georganta [3]

1 Department of Psychology, Northumbria University, Newcastle upon Tyne NE1 8ST, UK
2 School of Psychology, University of Leeds, Leeds LS2 9JT, UK; o.lainidi@leeds.ac.uk
3 Department of Psychology, University of Ioannina, 451 10 Ioannina, Greece; k.georganta@uoi.gr
* Correspondence: anthony.montgomery@northumbria.ac.uk

Abstract: Healthcare management faces significant challenges related to upward communication. Sharing information in healthcare is crucial to the improvement of person-centered, safe, and effective patient care. An adverse event (AE) is an unintended or unexpected incident that causes harm to a patient and may lead to temporary or permanent disability. Learning from adverse events in healthcare is crucial to the improvement of patient safety and quality of care. Informal communication channels represent an untapped resource with regard to gathering data about the development of AEs. In this viewpoint paper, we start by identifying how informal communication played a key factor in some high-profile adverse events. Then, we present three Critical Challenge points that examine the role of informal communication in adverse events by (1) understanding how the prevailing trends in healthcare will make informal communication more important, (2) explaining how informal communication is part of the group-level sensemaking process, and (3) highlighting the potential role of informal communication in "breaking the silence" around critical and adverse events. Gossip, as one of the most important sources of informal communication, was examined in depth. Delineating the role of informal communication and adverse events within the healthcare context is pivotal to understanding and improving team and upward communication in healthcare organizations. For clinical leaders, the challenge is to cultivate a climate of communication safety, whereby informal communication channels can be used to collect soft intelligence that are paths to improving the quality of care and patient safety.

Keywords: healthcare; informal communication; gossip; employee silence; patient safety

1. Introduction

Learning from adverse events (AEs) in healthcare is crucial to the improvement of person-centered, safe, and effective patient care. But, is there something that AEs are telling us that we are reluctant to learn? In the following paper, we begin by outlining the importance of informal communication in the following AEs: Mid-Staffordshire NHS Foundation Trust Public Inquiry, the case of Dr. Jayant Patel Bundaberg Hospital, Australia, the scandal at the Bristol Royal Infirmary, and the Lucy Letby scandal. The most common response to adverse events has been to increase the layers of formality to the healthcare process as a way to reduce the probability of critical events being missed. However, in this paper, we will argue that informal communication (which increases due to extra formality) should be our area of focus if we want to better understand how information is shared and communicated long before a critical point is reached. We will analyze informal communication via two very common and interrelated paths in healthcare—employee silence and gossip. We will argue that employee silence does not always equate with silence in the organization, and can find expression in the form of gossip that represents an 'early warning system' for adverse events [1]. The informal communication channels that individuals use are an untapped source of information about adverse events. Analyzing informal communication channels helps us understand the tension that exists between care and confidentially, which are the two key values in healthcare. We have structured the paper to outline what we can learn from adverse events, followed by an outline of three Critical Challenge points that can inform future research.

2. A Note on Definitions

Prior to beginning our discussion, a short note on definitions is warranted. Our discussion of adverse events will focus on the role of informal communication in healthcare settings, meaning "brief, more opportunistic interactions, taking place within and between different healthcare team members, as well as with a patient's family members or other caregivers" [2] (p. 289). Informal communication in work settings is defined as voluntary talk that does not have to be solely work- or task-focused [3]. There are different types of informal communication, but the present paper will explore the phenomenon of gossip in detail. Gossip is a form of informal communication "at the core of human social relationships" [4] (p. 811) and is defined as "the process of informally communicating value-laden information about members of a social setting" [5] (p. 25). Gossip occurs amongst at least two people and includes evaluative talk about those not present [6–9]. It is an informal way of communicating rules and establishing norms that lead to information and risk sharing [5]. Evaluations can be of either positive or negative valence and are more likely to be shared with members of the ingroup rather than the outgroup [10]. Senders and receivers report gossip with positive, negative, and neutral valence, each representing roughly a third of the gossip instances [11]; however, definitions generally do not attach valence or morality to its content or consequences [12–15]. Because the content of gossip can be both negative and positive, it has the potential to build both positive and negative social reputations [16–19].

Finally, sensemaking will be discussed throughout the paper. "Sensemaking involves the ongoing retrospective development of plausible images that rationalize what people are doing" [20] (p. 409). Moreover, efforts at sensemaking are more intense when the current state of the world is perceived to be different from the expected state of the world, which dovetails with the occurrence of AEs in healthcare. The emphasis in sensemaking on both understanding flux/chaos and the need to communicate makes it the perfect framework with which to disentangle employee silence and informal communication (i.e., gossip).

3. Adverse Events (AEs) and Informal Communication

An adverse event (AE) is an unintended or unexpected incident that causes harm to a patient and may lead to temporary or permanent disability [21]. Unless the protocol states otherwise, these must always be recorded on a case report form (CRF) and in the patient's medical notes. It is internationally recognized that 10–25% of healthcare episodes (in general hospitals, community hospitals, and general practice) are associated with an adverse event [22]. As learning from adverse events (AEs) is crucial to the improvement of person-centered, safe, and effective patient care [23], we draw upon examples of AEs to demonstrate how informal communication becomes an integral part of the sensemaking process [20] that, in some cases, can affect the decision to withhold concerns or speak up. We view informal communication as a collective attempt to make sense of problematic situations and what this can tell us about information sharing and transparency in the healthcare sector. Such communication is more likely to go under the radar and is more difficult to access in terms of research. Stress increases the likelihood of formal silence. There is significant evidence that healthcare education is building a culture of performance first, where individual well-being and asking difficult questions are far down the list of priorities [24]. A 'performance-first' culture does not encourage speaking up. Conversely, a 'performance-first' culture can encourage "speaking about" through gossip and informal conversations among colleagues, particularly when it comes to superiors and when speaking up against leaders is not an option.

Inquiries into the failings of care over time have found that, during the periods under investigation, the informal raising of concerns by many staff and managers about the level of care provided to patients was significantly increased [25]. For example, the Mid-Staffordshire Foundation NHS Trust failings of care highlighted how poor care was associated with the avoidable deaths of patients [26] (for details, see the Executive Summary of the Report of the Mid-Staffordshire NHS Foundation Trust Public Inquiry). The first report [27] clearly stated that there needed to be more openness and transparency throughout the trust, as, for example, incidents of poor patient care delivery were not formally recorded in the system or communicated to commissioners and regulators.

We know that the role of whistleblowing in exposing the failings and cover-ups was critical [28]. Before that, repetitive care declines were part of the employees' informal communications. The widespread disengagement in leadership responsibility addressed in the second report by Francis [29] describes failings and AEs of varying severity that can in no way go under the gossip radar [4]. The fact that the Francis report consists of two volumes suggests the magnitude and the multitude of AEs during the period under investigation. Unfortunately, informal communication routes in the forms of gossip and rumor around the series of failures, inadequacies, and cover-ups were not powerful enough to create a force to counteract what, in the Francis report, was named "negative culture" [29]. In their signals analysis paper, Carman et al. [30] highlighted how the content of informal communication amongst staff until May 2009 was indicative of what was happening, with employees discussing how they would not want their relatives and themselves to be patients. Thus, what employees informally talk about can be an important aspect of soft intelligence, a valuable resource with which to monitor how the day-to-day patient care is going, and probably a metric of care delivery quality—which means there are positive functions to gossip, as the pool of data related to what happens in the reality of the day-to-day delivery of patient care. The potential of gossip to be a necessary form of soft intelligence is highlighted by the recent typology of gossip by Lee and Barnes [31] into four categories, which include (a) protection-based gossip that alerts the workgroup to potential threats, (b) derogation-based gossip that negatively influences a coworker's reputation, (c) endorsement-based gossip that enhances a coworker's reputation through praise of exemplary behavior, and (d) communion-based gossip that strengthens interpersonal ties through social enjoyment. This approach is particularly relevant for adverse health and social care events in that it focuses on the behavior of consequence for the gossip sender's relationships with others.

The inquiry in the case of Dr. Jayant Patel at Bundaberg Hospital, Australia [32] can also provide insight into how employees responded to failings in patient care over time. Once again, the role of whistleblowing here was crucial. Still, an analysis of the events that led to the inquiry shows that collective sensemaking occurred before any whistleblowing decisions. On the level of informal communication, employees were unofficially discussing their concerns during the period of sensemaking, which led to either silence or formal reporting or whistleblowing [32]. When adverse events started occurring, employees engaged in discussions regarding Dr. Patel's behaviors, performance, and decisions amongst themselves since the first months after his arrival. We could hypothesize that these discussions—at that time, with no evidence and no severe AEs happening—can be classified as gossip, where a group of employees discussed Dr. Patel "behind his back". However, following the events that led to the formal inquiry (for details, see Edwards et al.) [32], it becomes more and more clear how the initial informal communication in the form of gossiping about the newly arrived surgeon is the unofficial attempt of the staff to make sense of decisions made by the hospital leaders. Testimonies provided by employees have indicated that Dr. Patel's behavior became a frequent topic of discussion. Edwards et al. [32] identified that those informal discussions were part of an attempt at "sensemaking" at this stage. While we do not imply any causal relationships between gossip and disclosure, it is possible that "keeping the gossip about Dr. Patel alive" for 24 months contributed to the external whistleblowing—after several attempts of official and unofficial reporting internally. The strategic benefit of temporarily remaining silent has been highlighted by Stouten et al. [33] in that it can serve several strategic functions, such as waiting for a more strategic time to act and allowing for time to form alliances to formulate an effective response.

Most recently, the Lucy Letby case has highlighted the problems inherent in a no-blame culture [34]. In 2023, Lucy Letby, a neonatal nurse, was sentenced to life in prison for the murder of seven babies and the attempted murder of six others. Much of the commentary on the case focused on the fact that concerns were raised by healthcare staff but ignored by managers [35]. The UK government has ordered an independent public inquiry into the circumstances surrounding the murders, so it is too early to reach any meaningful conclusions. However, the various reports surrounding the case reveals the importance of informal communication, such as "It was no secret that Letby was present when the infants suddenly collapsed, yet her crimes were so subtle they were imperceptible. Trainees started referring to her as "the angel of death", . . .". [36]. As noted by Leary [37], "success" in healthcare is measured by how much work is done, not how well the work is done. The Letby case, although arguably an outlier, is a reminder that the increased formalization of medical care is insufficient for gathering and hearing the important intelligence circulating in a hospital prior to an AE.

4. Understanding AEs via the Lens of Employee Silence/Voice

Healthcare workers frequently remain silent about work-related matters and prefer to use informal communication channels to share information. However, the evidence establishing the ubiquity of employee silence and voice in healthcare accounts largely for formal communication, upward communication channels, and speaking up to superiors and colleagues. The ongoing movement within healthcare towards standardizing procedures and digitalizing communications affirms that such informal routes of communication will become even more important. Accordingly, overburdened healthcare workers will continue seeking alternative ways to feel in control of their narratives and safely share sensitive information about work practices, and especially AEs.

Within the existing management practices, employee silence and voice are organizational behaviors that most frequently do not extend to informal communications between members of staff. In terms of our need to better understand AEs, this is lost data and a missed opportunity. For example, employees might be informally sharing their concerns in the form of venting or complaining about a colleague's or superior's behavior. When this is part of the "watercooler talk", it is likely to go under the radar as gossip rather than reach formal channels of communication and lead to change. In the event of an AE, staff can keep quiet while also informally discussing important issues (e.g., safety issues or unprofessional behaviors) amongst themselves or with family/friends through informal channels. Choosing gossip over a formal voice route can potentially function as a collective process of sensemaking [38,39] and discharge through the channels of informal communication among employees, when formal reporting is not considered an option. Viewing gossip as an alternative way to not staying silent can contribute to a better understanding of how and why employees might choose to withhold their voice or refrain from speaking up—especially when feeling unprotected from the consequences of doing so.

Employee silence/voice and gossip at work have been studied in parallel research domains. Still, considerable overlap exists, especially concerning events that challenge staff well-being and patient safety. Interest in workplace gossip endures because communication among colleagues is a vital source of informal communication within healthcare teams [40]. Additionally, studying all forms of communication in healthcare is critical given the relationship between effective communication between team members and improved patient safety and better healthcare delivery outcomes [41], increased self-reported employee well-being [42], lower self-reported burnout levels [43], and, overall, a more positive organizational culture [44].

Waddington [4] maintained that the negative view of gossip has overshadowed its potential value for healthcare organizations, with positive gossip often being linked to desired outcomes such as better social bonds within the team [45]. In this paper, we focus on the potential positive functions of gossip in relation to employee silence in healthcare, amidst crises and adverse events. Gossip, whether positive or negative, is anathema to systems pushing towards formalization and professionalization in healthcare. Obviously, getting everything (i.e., decision and opinion) on the record is desirable, but there is the distinct possibility that such approaches can make staff defensive and selective about what goes on the record [46]. The emphasis on informal communication stems from literature identifying the persistent problems found in formal communication channels [47], the limited availability of research reporting the effectiveness of speaking-up interventions in the sector [48], and the ubiquitous nature of employee silence in healthcare [49]. In the following, we present three Critical Challenge points with which to advance our understanding of gossip and employee silence in healthcare, by (1) understanding how the prevailing trends in healthcare will make informal communication more important, (2) explaining how informal communication is part of the group-level sensemaking process, and (3) highlighting the potential role of informal communication in "breaking the silence" around critical and adverse events.

5. Challenge Points

5.1. Challenge Point 1: Informal Communication Channels Will Become Increasingly Important in Healthcare

Healthcare professionals report experiencing high levels of work-related stress and are among the professions with the highest reported levels of burnout [50,51]. Burnout is linked to a culture of "performance-first", where mistakes are unwanted—even those that have minor implications for patient safety and quality of care, thus valorizing non-disclosure [49]. Moreover, healthcare organizations are constantly under formal scrutiny. Often, there is a tendency to attribute individual responsibility to the individual nurse and/or physician for suboptimal care delivery rather than identify organizational and systemic problems on a senior level [52,53]. This reality generates a culture of fear and blame, where everyone quickly becomes aware of the consequences of formal information sharing and speaking up. However, people need to share their thoughts and feelings, so informal sharing channels become an important outlet especially during intense events (e.g., AEs).

The workload and the demands of collaborating with many colleagues within and across teams expose healthcare professionals to a considerable amount of information related to day-to-day care, positive and negative events, concerns, and suspicions. This information overflow cannot only be managed via formal information-sharing channels due to this lack of trust. As informal communications are not likely to put healthcare professionals' jobs at stake and limit liability, informal communication (e.g., gossip) becomes the most viable option as a dynamic conversational event [54].

To achieve high-quality care, healthcare staff must communicate effectively both formally and informally [55]. Healthcare professionals collaborate with colleagues in both the same (e.g., nurses collaborating with nurses) and different specialties (e.g., nurses collaborating with doctors; doctors collaborating with allied professionals). Most often, clinical teams consist of members with different positions in the hierarchy. This can sometimes lead to communication complications that formal routes of transmission cannot always help resolve [2]. Taking into account excessive workloads, and constraints in time and resources, along with the need for practical solutions, healthcare staff often relies on the so-called "workarounds" [56], whereby the staff develops creative solutions to resource and staff shortages. Thus, there is an acceptance that being "silent" about the gaps in care is practical and solution-focused [57,58]. Workarounds present an interesting paradox. On the one hand, there may be an underlying driver of professional shaming that could help explain the silence around them. On the other hand, it is an organic response to silence (as opposed to apathy): because change will not ever be forthcoming, the problem needs to be "worked around" [59]. Thus, informal communication is often critical [2].

Congruently, attempts to include more formal channels of communication (i.e., computerized provider order entry, patient portal systems, and instant messaging apps) to overcome the communication barriers in healthcare have proven to be much less helpful than expected. These approaches tend to "formalize" communication at work, making it even more procedural, reserved, and planned, and potentially creating a work environment where employees feel every word is monitored [60]. Doing so seriously harms the spontaneity and the dynamic character of day-to-day work communications. Moreover, they lessen employees' feeling of control over their jobs, as aspects of their job become procedural, contributing to depersonalization and interpersonal distance between the team members [61].

Research has shown that informal communication among healthcare employees is positively linked to better support of the day-to-day needs and work demands of healthcare organizations [62,63]. Burm et al. [2] identified three valuable aspects of informal communication events in healthcare organizations: (1) a better sense of patients' baseline function; (2) a better understanding of the patient's needs, and (3) a better insight into the goals of care. Ward corridors and staff lounges are "knowledge-sharing venues", contributing to safer clinical practice and patient safety [64]. However, it is still unclear if all types of "informal chats" bring the same value in improving teamwork and quality of care. For example, studies recognize that informal interactions between nurses and non-physician professionals were positively linked with better collaborative care [65]. Conversely, informal interactions between nurses and physicians did not promote positive outcomes [66]. Accordingly, although informal communication is a valuable resource, there is not yet enough evidence indicating when and how it can better serve patient safety goals and quality of care.

In terms of informal communication routes, the extensively studied phenomenon of gossip is worthy of special consideration. According to Fan et al. [67], gossip is a fundamental part of every organization and not "just something that circulates within the confines of the organization". Baumeister et al. [68] have also discussed gossip as a mechanism for organizational learning with multiple functions, including information gathering, disseminating and validating, social enjoyment, and protecting one's group against norm violators [7,13,16,69]. Gossiping with colleagues can be beneficial in at least three ways on an individual level. Firstly, it is more economical in terms of time and resources to share information with a person who already understands the wider context—as opposed to gossiping with non-work friends. Secondly, gossiping generates reciprocal feelings of belonging and closeness when sharing information with colleagues [54], via its function as a bonding mechanism for social groups [13]. Thirdly, sharing sensitive information helps engender meaningful relationships beyond those dictated by the work role and fulfils the need for a "work confidant/work buddy" [70].

These three benefits suggest that gossip can be a pathway to meeting certain interpersonal and social needs in the workplace that formal communication pathways cannot adequately satisfy. When we view gossip through the lens of demanding healthcare environments, the importance of these benefits can be highlighted. The psychological and social needs of healthcare employees are most often neglected under the pressures of the day-to-day delivery of care, and employee well-being is not an operational priority for healthcare organizations and healthcare management. For example, during the COVID-19 pandemic, the Royal College of Nursing (RCN) and the British Medical Association (BMA) indicated unprecedented numbers of employees leaving, or considering leaving the field of healthcare, with psychological distress and burnout cited as main contributors [71–73].

Information in organizations is critical, and access to it is valuable. When information is not transparently shared using the formal channels of communication or not accessible to those who need it [10,74], employees will turn to informal routes, i.e., gossip [7]. Thus, gossip—in forms that do not contain false rumors, bullying intentions, or creating a toxic work environment—is a legitimate form of information exchange which requires for trust to be established to gain access to otherwise confidential information [70]. This means that the receivers of gossip information are considered ingroup members. We can see that the gossip content and the recipients of the information are chosen carefully, in the sense that the appropriate information is shared with the relevant people either because they will share the same opinions with the sender or they will be interested in the sender's evaluative comments [19]. In this sense, gossip may also contribute to workplace friendship and solidarity, especially when sharing sensitive information [14,70].

In organizations with a high power distance [75] and strict hierarchies [76], such as in healthcare, gossip can also protect employees from feeling powerless at a team level. Gossiping about toxic leaders, for example, has been identified to reduce the possibility of suffering from victimization [77]. When employees gossip about their leaders, they often feel better as gossip helps mitigate the effects of a bad leader's behavior; when the relationships between the employees are frequent and trusting, more negative gossip about the boss occurs [70]. Gossiping about the "boss" has been linked to cynical beliefs directed at supervisors, as well as the ways they make their decisions [78,79].

In the same vein, gossiping about a toxic leader can warn others or undermine the authority of poor managers [5], as it can function as a way of gathering reputational information that only direct observation allows [80,81]. Feldman [82] argued that gossip rests at the nexus of organizational power and politics. Kurland and Pelled [15] maintained that gossip is a means of acquiring power, highlighting the gain potential for groups lower in the hierarchy. Gossip in organizations is threatening to managers because it is almost impossible to control, as it flows via informal communication channels. Thus, such data are likely to be missed or ignored in AEs, but regularly feature as important in the official inquiries that follow tragic AEs. Healthcare organizations neglect gossip as a potential source of information regarding what is going on in the workplace, as well as the possibility that gossip is connected to the disclosure of important information. For example, in the Kerr/Haslam Inquiry, the investigation concerning the sexual abuse of psychiatric patients revealed that knowledge of these existed in informal channels of communication for over 20 years [4].

5.2. Challenge Point 2: Informal Communication Is Not Just "Cheap Talk"—It Is Part of the Group-Level Sensemaking Process

Informal communication, in the form of gossip, is pervasive in healthcare. As a phenomenon that occurs daily, gossip is part of daily work life, often mentioned as a "problem" in healthcare—especially due to the consequences of rumor and malicious gossip [4]. However, evidence suggests that not all gossip is linked to negative outcomes and that valence matters [14,45,83]. The full extent of gossip's benefits and whether they are more valuable to the workplace than its "dark side" has not been sufficiently explored and, despite the assumption that gossip is pervasive in healthcare, it has not been studied sufficiently concerning other prevailing organizational manifestations, such as burnout, work stress, or quality of care outcomes. We could speculate that formal communication in healthcare—which refers to scheduled events where the staff meets to discuss important topics, usually with a planned agenda (e.g., ward rounds, debriefings, or scheduled appointments with patients and their families) [2]—might be easier to research as opposed to informal communication.

Healthcare contexts have qualities and characteristics that are relatively stable and common across settings and countries [84]. Healthcare organizations thrive on gossip [4] due to complicated interpersonal dynamics within and across teams of diverse people [85]. Congruently, the need to gossip exists because many aspects are not discussed formally. The ubiquity of silence in healthcare sectors [86,87] suggests that there is a significant amount of information that never reaches the formal channels of communication. In times of crisis, informal conversations among trusted staff members are often related to "what is going wrong"; these conversations are a form of group-level sensemaking. Because organizational sensemaking is primarily a social activity, employees will check their interpretations via interacting with others, and then set the norms to act collectively [88]. Gossip is integral to sensemaking, which can lay the groundwork for sensegiving. In their role as sensegivers, line managers in health care have a symbolic role that goes beyond merely expressing values, and symbolic constructions are instrumental in creating meaning for others [89,90]. In sensemaking, gossip can inform new entrants to a profession about standards and appropriate behaviors expected at work, outline injunctive norms (i.e., rules for how not to behave), and serve as a model for well-established norms and regulations.

Gossip is strongly influenced by the context [91]. It emerges over the history of an organization [13], where it can help to establish and maintain important group norms and values [13,68]. In healthcare, it is critical that the context is taken into account, as, for example, regular handover meetings between shifts where formal and informal information is shared between colleagues [92]. Studies of conversations between colleagues are rare, but the existing data suggest that almost 50% of gossip is neither positive nor negative, but neutral [54,93]. Using neutral gossip adds weight to the idea that gossip serves important social functions beyond just information sharing. The COVID-19 pandemic resulted in the use of hybrid meetings, and we have little data yet on whether this hindered gossip. There is some initial evidence that informal communication is more likely to be neglected in remote work settings [94]. The lack of small talk afforded by virtual communication may have negatively impacted well-being, but this is an avenue for future research.

5.3. Challenge Point 3: The Role of Informal Communication in "Breaking the Silence" around Critical and Adverse Events

Informal communication will ramp up as crises develop, as individuals seek to make sense of a situation and line managers are under greater pressure to be sensegivers [95]. Within healthcare, gossip and rumor are attempts to process what is happening; as noted by Weick [20], "[o]rganizations talk in order to discover what they are saying, act in order to discover what they are doing". (p. 191). Congruently, although the content of gossip seems like an important factor, it is the context in which it occurs that is, in fact, the key [96]. Using informal chats fits the literature on voice cultivation within health care [97]. Underestimating gossip runs the risk of missing out on important sources of "soft intelligence" in health care. For example, Weick and Sutcliffe [20] highlight how, in the case of the Bristol Royal Infirmary, there was a continuation of a pediatric cardiac surgery program for almost 14 years despite the data showing a mortality rate roughly double the rate of any other center in England. We can only speculate as to the degree to which gossip among ancillary staff members had identified a serious problem, contrasted with the reported secrecy about doctors' performance and a lack of monitoring by management. The role of gossip in the extending or shortening of AEs is underresearched, but it is reasonable to suggest that instances of gossip may represent the early rumblings prior to the storms that accompany whistleblowing [1].

As noted by Leary [37], a workforce that must resort to whistleblowing is a symptom of a poor safety culture. Depending on whistleblowing to solve AEs is akin to waiting for a poorly functioning machine to explode. The formal silence that is characteristic of AEs finds expressions in informal routes. The interest in employee silence is entangled in the whistleblowing literature, as the latter represents the idea that a crisis point has been reached for the leadership and management in healthcare. Research and policies have focused on whistleblowing over the past four decades (for a literature review, see Blenkisopp et al. [98]). However, the interest in employee silence as a response to wrongdoings and patient-safety failures is much more recent. We know that employee silence in healthcare will likely go undetected until a breaking point is reached, and that it only sometimes results in whistleblowing [99]. Furthermore, most recent evidence highlights that speaking-up interventions in healthcare shows no significant impact on preventing or effectively resolving situations of employee silence [48]. Thus, the evidence suggests that employee silence in healthcare is shaped, maintained, and backed by pervasive "cultural forces" that characterize the healthcare sector across countries and continents. Accordingly, in healthcare organizations, employee silence can be an active form of behavior that can serve as the best strategy in particular situations, given the potential negative consequences of speaking up [100], indicating that treating silence as simply choosing not to speak up or as the opposite of speaking up [101] is too simplistic. Moreover, being silent in certain situations to avoid exposing colleagues could be considered a participative group climate—which is characterized by shared employee perceptions over what behaviors are more protective on the group level [102]. The behaviors mentioned above are likely to occur in healthcare where a culture of non-disclosure is valorized. Those lower in the hierarchy are less assertive and identify a knowledge gap between their superiors and themselves [49]. In essence, the early etiology of AEs in healthcare is characterized by staff talking internally but not sharing and being ignored, until exasperation is reached where the critical gossip finally reaches patients and families until a whistleblower bursts the bubble. Attaining a better balance between formal reporting and encouraging more talking among colleagues has the potential to prevent AEs and improve the quality of care.

In this paper, we have reviewed the role of information sharing in the development of AEs. The challenge for future research is (1) delineating how the soft intelligence provided via informal communication can be collected and used to prevent AEs, (2) identifying ways to better balance the inverse relationship between formalizing communication and defensive silence among staff, and (3) examining whether informal communication can be used to generate solutions to deal with the ubiquitous problem of employee silence.

6. Conclusions

Informal communication is important in healthcare. It serves important functions at the individual, group, and organizational levels. The ongoing movement within healthcare towards standardizing procedures and digitalizing communications within healthcare is likely to increase, and, thus, further overburden healthcare workers, who will seek alternative ways to feel in control of their narratives and safely share sensitive information about work practices. Informal communication can take many forms, but the phenomenon of gossip is worthy of special attention, given that it can allow staff to detect errors, reveal safety issues, and expose unethical behavior [103]. From a motivational perspective, gossiping can fulfil the self-determination theory's main elements [104], by making individuals feel more competent, in control, and more socially related to their colleagues. Doing so is consistent with a recent integrative review of workplace gossip, demonstrating that gossip serves four specific functions: information exchange, ego enhancement, social integration, and social segregation [105].

Gossip is worthy of greater consideration as an early-warning indicator of serious dysfunction in a healthcare organization. The reluctance of staff to share information outside their immediate team calls on us to understand why people with access to information feel a sense of togetherness with others who have the same access and a sense of separation from those who do not [106]. For example, improving feelings of psychological safety positively affects team effectiveness in healthcare units. Nevertheless, there is little or no literature on how different types of gossip (e.g., informal chats about events at work versus malicious gossip) influence team psychological safety. Interestingly, recent evidence suggests that the impact of psychological safety is more nuanced than previously assumed, whereby high levels of a psychological safety climate can actually harm the performance of routine tasks [107]. This is a reminder that linear assumptions of more always equaling better (e.g., more formal reporting or more psychological safety) is problematic. As noted by Weick [95], "[t]he veneer of rationality that overlies much talk about organizations tends to minimize the role of random activities". (p. 194). Line managers have a pivotal role to play in terms of listening for what is being talked about, but are faced with the challenge of how they can be in a position to ensure they hear such information.

Ultimately, we have an interesting tension between work policies that seek to further regulate the formal recording of work practices and procedures in contrast with the need for individuals to increase feelings of autonomy via informal communication paths such as gossip. We grow up with the admonishment that 'you shouldn't gossip', but maybe it is time for our healthcare leaders to change that to 'What are you gossiping about?'.

Author Contributions: A.M. and O.L. were responsible for the conceptualization and genesis of the paper. A.M., O.L. and K.G. were involved in writing—original draft preparation and writing—review and editing. All authors have read and agreed to the published version of the manuscript.

Funding: This research received no external funding.

Institutional Review Board Statement: Not applicable.

Informed Consent Statement: Not applicable.

Data Availability Statement: All data used are found within the manuscript.

Acknowledgments: We would like to thank Adrian Wilkinson & Wayne A. Hochwarter for their comments on an earlier draft of this paper.

Conflicts of Interest: The authors declare no conflicts of interest.

References

1. O'Connor, N.; Kotze, B.; Storm, V. What's to be done when 'foul whisp rings are abroad'? Gossip and rumour in health organisations. *Australas. Psychiatry* **2018**, *26*, 30–33. [CrossRef] [PubMed]
2. Burm, S.; Boese, K.; Faden, L.; DeLuca, S.; Huda, N.; Hibbert, K.; Goldszmidt, M. Recognising the importance of informal communication events in improving collaborative care. *BMJ Qual. Saf.* **2019**, *28*, 289–295. [CrossRef] [PubMed]
3. Fay, M.J. Informal communication of co-workers: A thematic analysis of messages. *Qual. Res. Organ. Manag. Int. J.* **2011**, *6*, 212–229. [CrossRef]
4. Waddington, K. Rethinking gossip and scandal in healthcare organizations. *J. Health Organ. Manag.* **2016**, *30*, 810–817. [CrossRef]
5. Noon, M.; Delbridge, R. News from behind my hand: Gossip in organizations. *Organ. Stud.* **1993**, *14*, 23–36. [CrossRef]
6. Eder, D.; Enke, J. The structure of gossip: Opportunities and constraints on collective expression among adolescents. *Am. Sociol. Rev.* **1991**, *56*, 494–508. [CrossRef]
7. Foster, E. Research on gossip: Taxonomy, methods, and future directions. *Rev. Gen. Psychol.* **2004**, *8*, 78–99. [CrossRef]
8. Taylor, G. Gossip as moral talk. In *Good Gossip*; Goodman, G., Ze'ev, A.B., Eds.; University Press of Kansas: Lawrence, KS, USA, 1994; pp. 34–446.
9. Michelson, G.; Van Iterson, A.; Waddington, K. Gossip in organizations: Contexts, consequences, and controversies. *Group Organ. Manag.* **2010**, *35*, 371–390. [CrossRef]
10. Wert, S.; Salovey, P. A social comparison account of gossip. *Rev. Gen. Psychol.* **2004**, *8*, 122–137. [CrossRef]
11. Dores Cruz, T.; Beersma, B.; Dijkstra, M.; Bechtoldt, M. The bright and dark side of gossip for cooperation in groups. *Front. Psychol.* **2019**, *10*, 1374. [CrossRef]
12. Brady, D.; Brown, D.; Liang, L. Moving beyond assumptions of deviance: The reconceptualization and measurement of workplace gossip. *J. Appl. Psychol.* **2017**, *102*, 1–25. [CrossRef]
13. Dunbar, R. Gossip: An evolutionary perspective. *Rev. Gen. Psychol.* **2004**, *8*, 100–110. [CrossRef]
14. Grosser, T.; Lopez-Kidwell, V.; Labianca, G. A social network analysis of positive and negative gossip in organizational life. *Group Organ. Manag.* **2010**, *35*, 177–212. [CrossRef]
15. Kurland, N.; Pelled, L. Passing the word: Toward a model of gossip and power in the workplace. *Acad. Manag. Rev.* **2000**, *25*, 428–438. [CrossRef]
16. Beersma, B.; Van Kleef, G. Why people gossip: An empirical analysis of social motives, antecedents, and consequences. *J. Appl. Soc. Psychol.* **2012**, *42*, 2640–2670. [CrossRef]
17. Feinberg, M.; Cheng, J.; Willer, R.; Guala, F. Gossip as an effective and low-cost form of punishment. *Behav. Brain Sci.* **2012**, *35*, 25. [CrossRef] [PubMed]
18. Zinko, R.; Rubin, M. Personal reputation and the organization. *J. Manag. Organ.* **2015**, *21*, 217–236. [CrossRef]
19. Van Iterson, A.; Waddington, K.; Michelson, G. Breaking the silence. The role of gossip in organizational culture. In *The Handbook of Organizational Culture and Climate*; Ashkanasy, N., Peterson, M., Wilderom, C., Eds.; Sage: Thousand Oaks, CA, USA, 2011; pp. 375–392.
20. Weick, K.; Sutcliffe, K.; Obstfeld, D. Organizing and the process of sensemaking. *Organ. Sci.* **2005**, *16*, 409–421. [CrossRef]
21. World Health Organization (WHO). *Glossary of Patient Safety Concepts and References. The Conceptual Framework for the International Classification for Patient Safety, Technical Annex, 2*; WHO: Geneva, Switzerland, 2009.
22. NHS Scotland. Learning from Adverse Events through Reporting and Review: A National Framework for NHS Scotland. 2016. Available online: https://www.healthcareimprovementscotland.org/our_work/governance_and_assurance/learning_from_adverse_events/national_framework.aspx (accessed on 11 January 2024).

23. Rafter, N.; Hickey, A.; Condell, S.; Conroy, R.; O'Connor, P.; Vaughan, D.; Williams, D. Adverse events in healthcare: Learning from mistakes. *QJM Int. J. Med.* **2015**, *108*, 273–277. [CrossRef] [PubMed]
24. Montgomery, A.; Lainidi, O. Understanding the link between burnout and sub-optimal care: Why should healthcare education be interested in employee silence? *Front. Psychiatry* **2022**, *13*, 818393. [CrossRef] [PubMed]
25. Barach, P.; Phelps, G. Clinical sensemaking: A systematic approach to reduce the impact of normalised deviance in the medical profession. *J. R. Soc. Med.* **2013**, *106*, 387–390. [CrossRef] [PubMed]
26. Kapur, N. Mid-Staffordshire Hospital and the Francis report: What does psychology have to offer? *Psychologist* **2014**, *27*, 16–20.
27. Francis, R. *Independent Inquiry into Care Provided by Mid-Staffordshire NHS Foundation Trust January 2005–March 2009*; The Stationery Office: London, UK, 2010; Volume 375.
28. Dyer, C. Francis report recommends a whistleblowing guardian in every NHS organisation. *BMJ* **2015**, *350*, h828. [CrossRef] [PubMed]
29. Francis, R. *Report of the Mid Staffordshire NHS Foundation Trust Public Inquiry: Executive Summary*; The Stationery Office: London, UK, 2013; Volume 947.
30. Carman, E.; Fray, M.; Waterson, P. Weak signals in healthcare: The case study of the Mid-Staffordshire NHS Foundation Trust. In *Congress of the International Ergonomics Association*; Springer: Cham, Switzerland, 2018; pp. 691–700.
31. Lee, S.; Barnes, C. An attributional process model of workplace gossip. *J. Appl. Psychol.* **2021**, *106*, 300–316. [CrossRef] [PubMed]
32. Edwards, M.; Lawrence, S.; Ashkanasy, N. How perceptions and emotions shaped employee silence in the case of "Dr. Death" at Bundaberg Hospital. In *Emotions and Organizational Governance*; Emerald Group Publishing Limited: Bingley, UK, 2016; Volume 12, pp. 341–379.
33. Stouten, J.; Tripp, T.; Bies, R.; De Cremer, D. When something is not right: The value of silence. *Acad. Manag. Perspect.* **2019**, *33*, 323–333. [CrossRef]
34. Mathew, R. Rammya Mathew: Lucy Letby and the limits of a no blame culture. *BMJ* **2023**, *382*, 1966. [CrossRef] [PubMed]
35. Dobson, J. We owe the families affected by Letby meaningful organisational change. *BMJ* **2023**, *382*, 1986. [CrossRef]
36. Halliday, J. 'Trust Me, I'm a Nurse': Why wasn't Lucy Letby Stopped as Months of Murder Went by? The Guardian. 2023. Available online: https://www.theguardian.com/uk-news/2023/aug/19/trust-me-im-a-nurse-why-wasnt-lucy-letbystopped-as-months-of-went-by (accessed on 2 February 2024).
37. Leary, A. Lessons not learned. *BMJ* **2023**, *382*, 1943. [CrossRef]
38. Waddington, K. Organisational gossip, sense-making and the spookfish: A reflexive account. *Int. J. Manag. Concepts Philos.* **2010**, *4*, 311–325. [CrossRef]
39. Fan, Z.; Dawson, P. Gossip as evaluative sensemaking and the concealment of confidential gossip in the everyday life of organizations. *Manag. Learn.* **2022**, *53*, 146–166. [CrossRef]
40. Altuntaş, S.; Şahin Altun, Ö.; Çevik Akyil, R. The nurses' form of organizational communication: What is the role of gossip? *Contemp. Nurse* **2014**, *48*, 109–116. [CrossRef]
41. Weaver, S.; Dy, S.; Rosen, M. Team-training in healthcare: A narrative synthesis of the literature. *BMJ Qual. Saf.* **2014**, *23*, 359–372. [CrossRef]
42. Ripp, J.; Peccoralo, L.; Charney, D. Attending to the emotional well-being of the health care workforce in a New York City health system during the COVID-19 pandemic. *Acad. Med.* **2020**, *95*, 1136–1139. [CrossRef]
43. Swensen, S.; Kabcenell, A.; Shanafelt, T. Physician-organization collaboration reduces physician burnout and promotes engagement: The Mayo Clinic experience. *J. Healthc. Manag.* **2016**, *61*, 105–127. [CrossRef]
44. Ratna, H. The importance of effective communication in healthcare practice. *Harv. Public Health Rev.* **2019**, *23*, 1–6. [CrossRef]
45. Thomas, S.; Rozell, E. Gossip and nurses: Malady or Remedy? *Health Care Manag.* **2007**, *26*, 111–115. [CrossRef]
46. Dixon-Woods, M.; Aveling, E.L.; Campbell, A.; Ansari, A.; Tarrant, C.; Willars, J.; Pronovost, P.; Mitchell, I.; Bates, D.W.; Dankers, C.; et al. What counts as a voiceable concern in decisions about speaking out in hospitals: A qualitative study. *J. Health Serv. Res. Policy* **2022**, *27*, 88–95. [CrossRef] [PubMed]
47. Karam, M.; Brault, I.; Van Durme, T.; Macq, J. Comparing interprofessional and interorganizational collaboration in healthcare: A systematic review of the qualitative research. *Int. J. Nurs. Stud.* **2018**, *79*, 70–83. [CrossRef] [PubMed]
48. Jones, A.; Blake, J.; Adams, M.; Kelly, D.; Mannion, R.; Maben, J. Interventions promoting employee "speaking-up" within healthcare workplaces: A systematic narrative review of the international literature. *Health Policy* **2021**, *125*, 375–384. [CrossRef] [PubMed]
49. O'Donovan, R.; McAuliffe, E. A systematic review exploring the content and outcomes of interventions to improve psychological safety, speaking up and voice behaviour. *BMC Health Serv. Res.* **2020**, *20*, 101. [CrossRef] [PubMed]
50. Prentice, S.; Dorstyn, D.; Benson, J.; Elliott, T. Burnout levels and patterns in postgraduate medical trainees: A systematic review and meta-analysis. *Acad. Med.* **2020**, *95*, 1444–1454. [CrossRef]
51. Salyers, M.; Bonfils, K.; Luther, L.; Firmin, R.; White, D.; Adams, E.; Rollins, A. The relationship between professional burnout and quality and safety in healthcare: A meta-analysis. *J. Gen. Intern. Med.* **2017**, *32*, 475–482. [CrossRef]
52. Ladher, N. End the culture of fear in healthcare. *BMJ* **2018**, *363*, k4467. [CrossRef]
53. Montgomery, A.; Panagopoulou, E.; Esmail, A.; Richards, T.; Maslach, C. Burnout in healthcare: The case for organisational change. *BMJ* **2019**, *366*, l4774. [CrossRef] [PubMed]

54. Begemann, V.; Lübstorf, S.; Meinecke, A.; Steinicke, F.; Lehmann-Willenbrock, N. Capturing workplace gossip as dynamic conversational events: First insights from Care Team Meetings. *Front. Psychol.* **2021**, *12*, 725720. [CrossRef] [PubMed]
55. McHugh, S.K.; Lawton, R.; O'Hara, J.K.; Sheard, L. Does team reflexivity impact teamwork and communication in interprofessional hospital-based healthcare teams? A systematic review and narrative synthesis. *BMJ Qual. Saf.* **2020**, *29*, 672–683. [CrossRef] [PubMed]
56. Lalley, C.; Malloch, K. Workarounds: The hidden pathway to excellence. *Nurse Lead.* **2010**, *8*, 29–32. [CrossRef]
57. Debono, D.S.; Greenfield, D.; Travaglia, J.F.; Long, J.C.; Black, D.; Johnson, J.; Braithwaite, J. Nurses' workarounds in acute healthcare settings: A scoping review. *BMC Health Serv. Res.* **2013**, *13*, 175. [CrossRef] [PubMed]
58. Mannion, R.; Exworthy, M.; Wiig, S.; Braithwaite, J. The power of autonomy and resilience in healthcare delivery. *BMJ* **2023**, *382*, e073331. [CrossRef] [PubMed]
59. Montgomery, A.; Lainidi, O.; Johnson, J.; Creese, J.; Baathe, F.; Baban, A.; Bhattacharjee, A.; Carter, M.; Dellve, L.; Doherty, E.; et al. Employee silence in health care: Charting new avenues for leadership and management. *Health Care Manag. Rev.* **2023**, *48*, 52–60. [CrossRef]
60. Chen, Y.; Tang, C.; Zhou, X.; Sarcevic, A.; Lee, S. Beyond formality: Informal communication in health practices. In Proceedings of the 2013 Conference on Computer Supported Cooperative Work Companion, San Antonio, TX, USA, 23–27 February 2013; pp. 307–312.
61. Califf, C.; Sarker, S.; Sarker, S. The bright and dark sides of technostress: A mixed-methods study involving healthcare IT. *MIS Q.* **2020**, *44*, 809–856. [CrossRef]
62. Conn, L.; Lingard, L.; Reeves, S.; Miller, K.; Russell, A.; Zwarenstein, M. Communication channels in general internal medicine: A description of baseline patterns for improved interprofessional collaboration. *Qual. Health Res.* **2009**, *19*, 943–953. [CrossRef] [PubMed]
63. Reeves, S.; Lewin, S. Interprofessional collaboration in the hospital: Strategies and meanings. *J. Health Serv. Res. Policy* **2004**, *9*, 218–225. [CrossRef] [PubMed]
64. Waring, J.J.; Bishop, S. "Water cooler" learning: Knowledge sharing at the clinical "backstage" and its contribution to patient safety. *J. Health Organ. Manag.* **2010**, *24*, 325–342. [CrossRef] [PubMed]
65. Redley, B.; Botti, M.; Wood, B.; Bucknall, T. Interprofessional communication supporting clinical handover in emergency departments: An observation study. *Australas. Emerg. Nurs. J.* **2017**, *20*, 122–130. [CrossRef] [PubMed]
66. Zwarenstein, M.; Rice, K.; Gotlib-Conn, L.; Kenaszchuk, C.; Reeves, S. Disengaged: A qualitative study of communication and collaboration between physicians and other professions on general internal medicine wards. *BMC Health Serv. Res.* **2013**, *13*, 494. [CrossRef] [PubMed]
67. Fan, Z.; Grey, C.; Kärreman, D. Confidential gossip and organization studies. *Organ. Stud.* **2021**, *42*, 1651–1664. [CrossRef]
68. Baumeister, R.; Zhang, L.; Vohs, K. Gossip as cultural learning. *Rev. Gen. Psychol.* **2004**, *8*, 111–121. [CrossRef]
69. Emler, N. Gossip, reputation, and adaptation. In *Good Gossip*; Goodman, R., Ze, A.B., Eds.; University of Kansas Press: Lawrence, KS, USA, 1994; pp. 34–46.
70. Ellwardt, L.; Wittek, R.; Wielers, R. Talking about the boss: Effects of generalized and interpersonal trust on workplace gossip. *Group Organ. Manag.* **2012**, *37*, 521–549. [CrossRef]
71. BMA. The Mental Health and Wellbeing of the Medical Workforce-Now and beyond COVID-19. 2020. Available online: https://www.bma.org.uk/media/2475/bma-covid-19-andnhs-staff-mental-health-wellbeing-report-may-2020.pdf (accessed on 11 January 2024).
72. BMA. *Moral Distress and Moral Injury: Recognising and Tackling It for UK Doctors*; British Medical Association: London, UK, 2021.
73. Royal College of Nursing (2020), Building a Better Future for Nursing: RCN Members Have Their Say. Available online: https://www.rcn.org.uk/professional-development/publications/rcn-builiding-a-better-future-covid-pub009366 (accessed on 11 January 2024).
74. Michelson, G.; Mouly, V. 'You didn't hear it from us but...': Towards an understanding of rumour and gossip in organisations. *Aust. J. Manag.* **2002**, *27*, 57–65. [CrossRef]
75. Krishnakumar, D.; Caskey, R.; Hughes, A. Examining the influence of power distance on psychological safety within healthcare teams. In Proceedings of the International Symposium on Human Factors and Ergonomics in Health Care, Virtual, 12–16 April 2021; SAGE Publications: Los Angeles, CA, USA, 2021; Volume 10, No. 1. pp. 194–198.
76. Bate, P. Changing the culture of a hospital: From hierarchy to networkedcommunity. *Public Adm.* **2000**, *78*, 485–512. [CrossRef]
77. Silverman, S.; Johnson, R.; McConnell, N.; Carr, A. Arrogance: A formula for leadership Failure. *Ind. -Organ. Psychol.* **2012**, *50*, 21–28.
78. Kouzes, J.; Posner, B. *The Student Leadership Practices Inventory (LPI): The Facilitator's Guide*; Wiley: New York, NY, USA, 2005; Volume 61.
79. Pelletier, K.; Bligh, M. The aftermath of organizational corruption: Employee attributions and emotional reactions. *J. Bus. Ethics* **2008**, *80*, 823–844. [CrossRef]
80. Bozoyan, C.; Vogt, S. The impact of third-party information on trust: Valence, source, and reliability. *PLoS ONE* **2016**, *11*, e0149542. [CrossRef] [PubMed]
81. Burt, R.; Knez, M. Trust and third-party gossip. In *Trust in Organizations: Frontiers of Theory and Research*; Kramer, R., Tyler, T., Eds.; Sage: Thousand Oaks, CA, USA, 1996; pp. 68–89.

82. Feldman, S. Secrecy, information, and politics: An essay on organizational decision making. *Hum. Relat.* **1988**, *41*, 73–90. [CrossRef]
83. Waddington, K.; Fletcher, C. Gossip and emotion in nursing and healthcare organizations. *J. Health Organ. Manag.* **2005**, *19*, 378–394. [CrossRef] [PubMed]
84. Pope, R. Organizational Silence in the NHS: 'Hear no, See no, Speak no'. *J. Chang. Manag.* **2019**, *19*, 45–66. [CrossRef]
85. Baltimore, J.J. Nurse collegiality: Fact or fiction? *Nurs. Manag.* **2006**, *37*, 28–36. [CrossRef]
86. Lainidi, O.; Jendeby, M.K.; Montgomery, A.; Mouratidis, C.; Paitaridou, K.; Cook, C.; Johnson, J. An integrative systematic review of employee silence and voice in healthcare: What are we really measuring? *Front. Psychiatry* **2023**, *14*, 1111579. [CrossRef]
87. Mannion, R.; Davies, H. Cultures of silence and cultures of voice: The role of whistleblowing in healthcare organisations. *Int. J. Health Policy Manag.* **2015**, *4*, 503–505. [CrossRef]
88. Maitlis, S.; Christianson, M. Sensemaking in organizations: Taking stock and moving forward. *Acad. Manag. Ann.* **2014**, *8*, 57–125. [CrossRef]
89. Gioia, D.; Chittipeddi, K. Sensemaking and sensegiving in strategic change initiation. *Strateg. Manag. J.* **1991**, *12*, 433–448. [CrossRef]
90. Parzefall, M.; Jacqueline, A. Making sense of psychological contract breach. *J. Manag. Psychol.* **2011**, *26*, 12–27. [CrossRef]
91. Mills, C. Experiencing gossip: The foundations for a theory of embedded organizational gossip. *Group Organ. Manag.* **2010**, *35*, 213–240. [CrossRef]
92. Tobiano, G.; Ting, C.; Ryan, C.; Jenkinson, K.; Scott, L.; Marshall, A. Front-line nurses' perceptions of intra-hospital handover. *J. Clin. Nurs.* **2020**, *29*, 2231–2238. [CrossRef] [PubMed]
93. Robbins, M.; Karan, A. Who gossips and how in everyday life? *Soc. Psychol. Personal. Sci.* **2020**, *11*, 185–195. [CrossRef]
94. Blanchard, A. The effects of COVID-19 on virtual working within online groups. *Group Process. Intergroup Relat.* **2021**, *24*, 290–296. [CrossRef]
95. Weick, K. *Making Sense of the Organization*; Blackwell: Oxford, UK, 2001.
96. Bergmann, J. *Discreet Indiscretions: The Social Organization of Gossip*; Gruyter: New York, NY, USA, 1993.
97. Satterstrom, P.; Kerrissey, M.; DiBenigno, J. The voice cultivation process: How team members can help upward voice live on to implementation. *Adm. Sci. Q.* **2021**, *66*, 380–425. [CrossRef]
98. Blenkinsopp, J.; Snowden, N.; Mannion, R.; Powell, M.; Davies, H.; Millar, R.; McHale, J. Whistleblowing over patient safety and care quality: A review of the literature. *J. Health Organ. Manag.* **2019**, *33*, 737–756. [CrossRef]
99. Knoll, M.; Van Dick, R. Do I hear the whistle...? A first attempt to measure four forms of employee silence and their correlates. *J. Bus. Ethics* **2013**, *113*, 349–362. [CrossRef]
100. Creese, J.; Byrne, J.; Matthews, A.; McDermott, A.; Conway, E.; Humphries, N. "I feel I have no voice": Hospital doctors workplace silence in Ireland. *J. Health Organ. Manag.* **2021**, *35*, 178–194. [CrossRef] [PubMed]
101. Sherf, E.; Parke, M.; Isaakyan, S. Distinguishing voice and silence at work: Unique relationships with perceived impact, psychological safety, and burnout. *Acad. Manag. J.* **2021**, *64*, 114–148. [CrossRef]
102. Lee, G.L.; Diefendorff, J.M.; Kim, T.Y.; Bian, L. Personality and participative climate: Antecedents of distinct voice behaviors. *Hum. Perform.* **2014**, *27*, 25–43. [CrossRef]
103. Waddington, K. *Gossip, Organization and Work: A Research Overview*; Routledge: Oxon, UK, 2022.
104. Deci, E.; Olafsen, A.; Ryan, R. Self-determination theory in work organizations: The state of a science. *Annu. Rev. Organ. Psychol. Organ. Behav.* **2017**, *4*, 19–43. [CrossRef]
105. Sun, T.; Schilpzand, P.; Liu, Y. Workplace gossip: An integrative review of its antecedents, functions, and consequences. *J. Organ. Behav.* **2023**, *44*, 311–334. [CrossRef]
106. Bingley, W.; Greenaway, K.; Haslam, S. A social-identity theory of information-access regulation (SITIAR): Understanding the psychology of sharing and withholding. *Perspect. Psychol. Sci.* **2022**, *17*, 827–840. [CrossRef]
107. Eldor, L.; Hodor, M.; Cappelli, P. The limits of psychological safety: Nonlinear relationships with performance. *Organ. Behav. Hum. Decis. Process.* **2023**, *177*, 104255. [CrossRef]

healthcare

MDPI

Opinion

What Is Truly Informed Consent in Medical Practice and What Has the Perception of Risk Got to Do with It?

Catherine Jane Calderwood [1], Geir Sverre Braut [2] and Siri Wiig [3,*]

[1] Faculty of Science, University of Strathclyde, Glasgow G1 1XQ, UK; catherine.calderwood@strath.ac.uk
[2] Stavanger University Hospital, N-4068 Stavanger, Norway; geir.sverre.braut@sus.no
[3] SHARE—Centre for Resilience in Healthcare, Faculty of Health Sciences, University of Stavanger, N-4036 Stavanger, Norway
* Correspondence: siri.wiig@uis.no

Abstract: Making decisions about risk, describing and appropriately explaining risk in medical practice is complex for patients and professionals. In this paper, we investigate how the concept of consent is practiced differently in the UK and Norway and discuss pros and cons of the chosen approaches from a patient safety culture perspective. We argue that consent is a fundamental part of the safety culture and influence on health system functioning and patient and staff safety. Examples from the UK and Norway are used and discussed in terms of how risk perception influences consent processes and practices.

Keywords: consent; patient safety culture; risk; risk perception; compensation

1. Introduction

Risk is fundamentally complex in medical practice, and medical practice involves the risk of patient harm and complications. Making decisions about risk, describing and appropriately explaining risk are more complex still—for patients and professionals. The perception of risk has many facets [1]. Professionals are expected to be up to date with the latest research, facts and figures, guidelines, and rapidly changing information whilst working in a highly pressured clinical role. For the patient, their perception of risk, preferences, and willingness to accept risk can be based on their own values, their past experience, the health dilemma presented, and how it is impacting on their life, their understanding, and interest, whether the stakes are large or small. How should knowledge about risk be communicated to the patient? How should patient preferences be considered and integrated in shared decision-making processes? What level of risk is acceptable not to explain? How much does fear of litigation and a culture of blame drive the process, and do different legal systems influence clinical practice? To exemplify, Table 1 shows the diversity in understanding and talking about risk and how this may play out in practice based on a real-life clinical situation.

As exemplified above, there are numerous layers when we talk about risk and risk perception and how people, patients, and professionals perceive, balance, and weight different information [1]. They relate to individual needs, competences, and preferences; they relate to cultural traits and attitudes of how patient safety is conceptualised in a system, unit, or in terms of individual responsibility and who is responsible, accountable, and to blame; they relate to the role of the treatment indication for professionals compared to decision-making for the patient concerning the available treatment, alternatives, and evidence; and they relate to contextual settings and regulatory frameworks in different healthcare systems. In health care, making decisions about risk and if and how to intervene happen in the relationship between the professionals and the patients and happen many times on a daily basis. This implies informing and consenting as a core element in health care [2,3]. However, we may question whether consenting is core in the patient safety culture debate and whether it should be? Or does this field focus more on structural and cultural elements in how systems are set up to prevent and respond to adverse events. However, when poor outcomes occur, one will turn to medical records to see what happened during the consultation and treatment process, and how well patients were informed about the risks, possible benefits, likelihood, and consequences, whether they consented based on sufficient information, and also whether they had the capacity to consent. There is not necessarily a link between patient safety measures, informed consent, and the patient safety culture, but this is a highly dynamic field with a continuous need for an ongoing debate to keep up with new developments, risks, and demands from different parties.

In this paper we aim to pick up this debate and draw on how the concept of consent is practiced differently in the UK and Norway and discuss pros and cons of the chosen approaches from a patient safety culture perspective. We argue that consent is a fundamental part of the safety culture and influence on health system functioning and patient and staff safety. This will be illustrated based on examples from the UK and Norway, and discussed in terms of how risk perception could influence this and how compensation schemes are set up and could potentially play a role in medical decision-making either in a defensive or risk-seeking direction. Risk perception may be amplified or attenuated based on socio-cultural elements and structures in any healthcare system [1] and should be placed higher on the agenda when we try to understand the role of consent and how it relates to safety culture. Diverse risk perception between patients and professionals may exist, but the ability to influence decisions may vary between professionals and across cultural settings and norms.

Table 1. Clinical example of risk-based decisions.

Making Decisions Based on Risk in Maternity Services
As a practising obstetrician, first author CC was once counselling 2 women in succession who had screening for genetic abnormalities in early pregnancy. The arbitrary cut-off for informing women of a 'high-risk' result is that the risk of the baby being affected is greater than 1 in 150. This cut-off was simply determined statistically as encompassing 5% of women who were screened. No other scientific, clinical, moral, ethical, or other considerations are involved. All other women were informed that they had a 'low-risk' result. The first woman had not been notified but had requested to see her results. These showed a risk of an affected baby of 1 in 400. She proceeded to a definite diagnostic test (which itself carried a risk of an adverse outcome of 0.5%) as she did not want to tolerate any uncertainty. The next woman had a 'high-risk' result of 1 in 10. This level of risk is very unusual, and CC assumed (as with most women with a high-risk result) that she would proceed to a definitive test. However, she asked 'but doctor this means there's a 90% chance the baby will be ok?'. Yes was replied and she left the room without further intervention.

2. Informed Consent—What Is It?

By 'informed consent', we mean the process of providing patients with sufficient information to enable them to make a voluntary and informed decision regarding whether to undergo a procedure or not, and that the patients are able to understand the information given [4]. Consent from the patient must be obtained for all interactions, e.g., an examination, a blood test, an onward referral. This may be oral, written, or implied—such as when a patient offers their arm for a requested blood test. European countries have differing expectations and guidance when it comes to informed consent for operative or invasive procedures—some require written informed consent (e.g., the UK), while others inform but do not obtain patients' consent in a written format (e.g., Norway). Does it matter?

The literature shows that from the patients' perspective, consent forms may fall short of providing information to inform decision-making. They may be too complex and difficult to read and comprehend; hence, the patient–doctor conversation is recognised for its importance [5]. From a medical point of view, how doctors inform and ensure patients are provided with sufficient information and making sure they understand it is a fundamental part of medical practice. This relates to how they are culturally and socially influenced in their risk understanding, or risk-seeking or risk-averse behaviour in decision-making processes. The need for balancing information provision, tailoring information, and assessing patients' competence and literacy level, with an increasingly more up-to-date and healthcare-literate population with access to medical information online may challenge this information and consent process for clinicians.

3. Principles and Practice for Informed Consent in the UK and Norway

In the Norwegian legislation on patient's rights, it is stated that health care, as a rule, shall be based upon a "valid consent" from the person concerned, as stated in Section 4.1 in the Patients' Rights Act. The concept of valid consent should be interpreted in a wider context than "informed consent" [6]. In addition to sufficient information being given, the patient must be cognitively capable of understanding the implications and there must be real freedom to refuse accepting the care offered. This puts an obligation upon health professionals to ensure that the patient has a minimum understanding of the risk following the suggested intervention and the risk related to not accepting the offered services. The Act also states that if the patient withdraws their consent, information shall be given on the possible consequences of such a decision.

There are only a few situations where written consent is practiced and required by law. These are prenatal diagnostics, sterilisation, altruistic organ donation, genetic therapies, and assisted fertilisation, chosen in particular because they are not deemed an 'essential medical intervention or care'. In all other cases, conversation and discussion regarding surgery and intervention is recorded in the case notes according to the legal requirements but neither the patient nor the practitioner sign a document.

In the UK, guidance for shared decision-making and informed consent was updated by the General Medical Council in November 2020 [7]. This followed the high-profile case of a pregnant woman, Nadine Montgomery, who had diabetes. Due to complications during his birth more than 20 years ago, her son has significant disability and lifelong care needs. In the Montgomery court case in 2015 [8], the court ruled that if Ms Montgomery had been made aware of all the possible risks of a vaginal birth, she would have chosen a caesarean section. For the first time, this put the patient rather than the professional in the 'driving seat' regarding how much information and detail of risk should be given and how informed consent should be obtained. Table 2 [7] (p. 5) illustrates what are considered the seven principles for shared decision-making and informed consent from this document.

Table 2. Principles for informed consent [7] (p. 5).

Principle	Description
1	All patients have the right to be involved in decisions about their treatment and care and be supported to make informed decisions if they are able.
2	Decision-making is an ongoing process focussed on meaningful dialogue: the exchange of relevant information specific to the individual patient.
3	All patients have the right to be listened to, and to be given the information they need to make a decision and the time and support they need to understand it.
4	Doctors must try to find out what matters to patients so they can share relevant information about the benefits and harms of proposed options and reasonable alternatives, including the option to take no action.
5	Doctors must start from the presumption that all adult patients have capacity to make decisions about their treatment and care. A patient can only be judged to lack capacity to make a decision at a specific time, and only after assessment in line with legal requirements.
6	The choice of treatment or care for patients who lack capacity must be of overall benefit to them, and decisions should be made in consultation with those close to them or advocating for them.
7	Patients whose right to consent is affected by law should be supported to be involved in the decision-making process, and to exercise choice if possible.

In points 6 and 7 above, capacity is described as decision-specific and time-specific; so, a person can only have capacity or lack capacity to make a specific decision at a specific time. Each jurisdiction of the UK has its own mental capacity legislation which, together with accompanying codes of practice, provides a framework for making decisions when patients lack the capacity to decide for themselves.

In the UK, the legal need for informed consent is described in the Health and Social Care Act 2008 Regulations. It is standard procedure for surgical operations and invasive procedures and interventions to require written consent from the patient. However, the GMC guidance states: 'Obtaining a patient's consent needn't always be a formal, time-consuming process. While some interventions require a patient's signature on a form, for most healthcare decisions, you can rely on a patient's verbal consent, as long as you are satisfied they've had the opportunity to consider any relevant information and decided to go ahead. Although a patient can give consent verbally (or non-verbally) you should make sure this is recorded in their notes [7] (p. 9)'.

Despite the rhetoric that the signature is hugely significant, the reality is that consent should be a process with two-way dialogue, as above, and many UK doctors would also be surprised at the actual GMC wording regarding the consent form [7]. 'Consent forms can be a helpful prompt to share key information, as well as a standard way to record a decision that can make regular review easier. Consent forms can also be used to review decisions made at an earlier stage, and the relevant information they were based on. But, filling in a consent form isn't a substitute for a meaningful dialogue tailored to the individual patient's needs'.

The use of standardised consent forms with pre-printed information to reduce variation and increase accuracy has followed on from the Montgomery case. Giving people the opportunity to consider their options over a period of time, with information to take home to discuss with family and their General Practitioner (GP), is sometimes offered.

Generic forms are provided to try to ensure all aspects of significant risk are disclosed and this is obviously dependent on the nature of the procedure being proposed. The benefits, alternatives, and unexpected procedures that may be required during the operation are flagged and patient opinion is sought as well as highlighting the option of doing nothing. A recent study has shown the improved accuracy and reduced omission error rate when consent is obtained using a digital form, and importantly, this also improved the patient experience of shared decision-making [9]. Practitioners believe this ensures fully informed consent, protecting both the patient and doctor. This practice is not universal, although it is increasing. Inevitably, differences in knowledge, experience, time constraints, complexity level, and individual patient characteristics will lead to variation. Of course, as most procedures end without harm, these processes are not further examined in the vast majority of cases, in contrast to when there is an adverse outcome. Also worth noting is when harm occurs, a lack of information and lack of communication may add a burden to the problematic situation for the patient and their families.

As described, the Norwegian and UK practices are different. However, the requirements for informing patients about the risk associated with the relevant procedure and involving patients in the decision-making process is equally as important in both countries.

4. Compensation Schemes from Medical Harm

Routes for compensation are very different in the two countries. Norwegian legislation clearly defines right and duties for informing and making decisions with patients. The Norwegian System of Patient Injury Compensation (NPE)—a government-funded compensation scheme—allows complaints to be brought forward by the patient in an application for compensation after possibly being harmed. In cases where patients experience financial loss as a result of an injury caused by insufficient medical treatment, compensation will be approved if the application fulfils specific conditions [10]. As a patient, you are, in principle, entitled to receive economic compensation if you suffer a harm caused by a failure in the provision of health care, even if nobody is to blame, and you have or probably will experience economic losses due to this harm. The complaint is, in the first instance, considered by legal and medical officers in the NPE, who decide whether there has been substandard care and award a level of compensation that is determined by the level of harm caused and the long-term needs of the patient. The decision made by the NPE can be brought forward to an expert panel for review and a final decision if the patient is not content with the decision in the first instance.

This compensation scheme is funded by public taxes and the handling of cases is accessible at no cost to all of the Norwegian population. The providers of health care in Norway, public as well as private, are obliged by law to take part in this system, and according to specific regulations, also have to pay an annual fee for participation. Every provider of health care is also obliged to give information to the NPE so that the cases may be investigated. Apart from this, the care providers, either individuals or institutions, have no other obligations, e.g., related to meeting with a panel or being available for oral questioning. The legal parts in this system are merely the "public" represented by the NPE and the single patient. Information given to the NPE will not usually be used in the investigation of the practice of individual healthcare professionals, neither by the supervisory board nor the police.

In the UK, there is no such overall scheme at no cost to patients. Individual patients can, through the legal system, make a claim for compensation if harm has occurred and can be proven. Legal and other costs are incurred by the individual and may be recouped if the case is successful. Compensation is paid from NHS resources. Patients may receive compensation for injury, and also for loss of work and future earnings, and for costs of long-term care. Professionals have indemnity provided via their NHS employer. The Montgomery case marked a shift away from the previous legal test of duty of care, which was that the healthcare practitioner must have acted in a way that fell short of acceptable professional standards. Known as the 'Bolam' principle, this tested whether the actions of the health professional in question could be supported by a 'responsible body of clinical opinion'. Thus, the individual's practice was examined to apportion blame and prove negligence regardless of systemic failures. Montgomery has changed the context for consent from the position of the clinician to that of the patient.

5. Discussion

How do we achieve truly informed consent in a fast-paced system with demands on time and resources, and should or does legal practice have influence? What is certain is that optimizing shared decision-making and truly informed consent is best practice and should be at the core of healthcare interactions. Up until now, conversations about risk and options regarding procedures have been in the domain of individual practitioners with a relationship with their patients. Recent progress has been made towards standardizing information given to patients and to ensuring that this is timely, at an appropriate level, and that patients and their families understand the options. It is clear than even in outwardly similar European countries, the compensation schemes for harm in health care are markedly different, and even what would appear to be the simplest of interventions—signing or not signing a consent form—are not acknowledged as necessary in both systems. The responsibility of an individual working in a complex healthcare system also opens up a very interesting debate. Compensation schemes have evolved differently and several proposals for 'no blame' schemes in the UK have been considered and debated, so far unsuccessfully, in recent times.

Compensation schemes are not necessarily connected with the principles and practice related to informed consent. However, a system requiring evidence of guilt as a prerequisite for compensation will invite to establishing formalised and strict procedures to document the agreed terms and information provided between the patient and the care provider.

The major difference between Norway and the UK from a patient safety culture perspective relates to the UK mandatory written consent and compensation claims handled in the legal system when fault or negligence by an individual is often found; while Norway has established a compensation system outside if the legal court system, individual practitioners are not held to account with regard to financial compensation, and in most cases do not practice obtaining written consent. This does not mean one of the systems is better than the other, or that some patients are better informed with either approach. However, we argue this needs more attention as resources will most likely be more constrained in the future, patients will be more informed, and technological solutions and artificial intelligence will contribute to pushing the boundaries of knowledge and medical treatment options. Still, doctors and patients are the ones who need to make decisions and consent to treatment and care based on the available information.

6. Conclusions

What, therefore, is truly informed consent? As discussed, the challenges of understanding risk, describing risk, managing uncertainty and personal values, and views and preferences (variable between both patients and professionals, of course) are complex and layered [11]. In the UK, the need for written consent is seen as a safeguard for both parties, but in reality, the requirements for informed consent are the same in both countries. The patient should be enabled to understand the risks involved in health care, source information relevant to them, and accept treatment with as much appropriate knowledge as possible. This also includes patients with low health literacy, resources, and abilities to communicate. In 'safety' terms, the fundamentals of good communication, respect for the individual, and involvement in decisions are a necessity. The ability of the patient to speak up if these fundamentals are not met for them is fundamental, but often proves difficult in practice for many practical reasons. Until now, consent has not, we believe, been part of the patient safety 'culture', integrated in training and teaching and good work practice and discussed in the literature. During the scrutiny that comes after an adverse event, the fundamental principles of informed decision-making and consent are carefully examined. However, we may question whether this aspect of safety, which is of course the only aspect the patient has any control over, has received the due diligence and input it rightly deserves. Further attention is needed to enable continuous reflection for professionals and regulators. The field is changing rapidly as access to information and technological advancement will play a key role in future healthcare provision and decision-making

7. Future Directions

We would all want to be fully informed in order to understand the risks and options we may have as patients, and also the possible decision to say no and do nothing. This is an ongoing debate in many counties [12,13] and if 10% of all health care causes harm [14], comprehensive information should be front and centre of how the present-day safety culture matures. This may lead to patients deciding not to have any treatment at all. The elements of risk, perception, uncertainty, and consent should be more strongly integrated in the future patient safety culture debate to enable sound discussions and decision-making in healthcare provision.

Author Contributions: Author C.J.C. had the idea together with S.W. C.J.C. drafted the first version of the manuscript followed by significant input and contributions from G.S.B. and S.W. All authors have read and agreed to the published version of the manuscript.

Funding: The authors received no funding.

Institutional Review Board Statement: Not applicable.

Informed Consent Statement: Not applicable.

Data Availability Statement: Not relevant.

Conflicts of Interest: The authors declare no conflicts of interest.

References

1. Pidgeon, N.; Kasperson, R.E.; Slovic, P. *The Social Amplification of Risk*; Cambridge University Press: Cambridge, UK, 2003.
2. Kovic, Ž.; Kobua, M.; Fogarty, M.; Donohoe, C.L.; Kelly, M.E.; Fitzmaurice, G.J.; Fitzgerald, M.; Zambra, P.; Geary, U.; Ward, M.E. Valid consent in the acute hospital setting: Perspectives of patients and members of the public. *Ir. J. Med. Sci.* **2024**, *193*, 1703–1714. [CrossRef] [PubMed]
3. Vansweelt, T.; Glover-Thomas, N. (Eds.) *Informed Consent and Health. A Global Analysis*; Global Perspectives on Medical Law series; Elgar Online: Cheltenham, UK, 2020.
4. Villanueva, C.; Talwar, A.; Doyle, M. Improving informed consent in cardiac surgery by enhancing preoperative education. *Patient Educ. Couns.* **2018**, *101*, 2047–2053. [CrossRef] [PubMed]
5. Manta, C.; Ortiz, J.; Moulton, B.; Sonnad, S. From the Patient Perspective, Consent Forms Fall Short of Providing Information to Guide Decision Making. *J. Patient Saf.* **2021**, *17*, e149–e154. [CrossRef] [PubMed]
6. Syse, A. Norway: Valid (as opposed to informed) consent. *Lancet* **2000**, *356*, 1347–1348. [CrossRef] [PubMed]

7. General Medical Council. *Decision Making and Consent*. 2020. Available online: https://www.gmc-uk.org/-/media/documents gmc-guidance-for-doctors---decision-making-and-consent-english_pdf-84191055.pdf (accessed on 3 August 2024).
8. Montgomery v Lanarkshire Health Board [2015] SC 11 [2015] 1 AC 1430. Available online: https://www.supremecourt.uk/cases docs/uksc-2013-0136-judgment.pdf (accessed on 3 August 2024).
9. Dyke, R.; St-John, E.; Shah, H.; Walker, J.; Loughran, D.; Anakwe, R.; Nathwani, D. Comparing shared decision making using paper and digital consent process. A multi-site, single centre study in a trauma and orthopaedic department. *Surgeon* **2023**, 2 235–241. [CrossRef] [PubMed]
10. Wiig, S.; Macrae, C.; Frich, J.; Øyri, S.F. Naming the "baby" or the "beast"? The importance of concepts and labels in healthcar safety investigation. *Front. Public Health* **2023**, *11*, 1087268. [CrossRef] [PubMed]
11. van der Pijl, M.S.G.; Klein Essink, M.; van der Linden, T.; Verweij, R.; Kingma, E.; Hollander, M.H.; De Jonge, A.; Verhoeven, C. Consent and refusal of procedures during labour and birth: A survey among 11 418 women in the Netherlands. *BMJ Qual. Saf* **2024**, *33*, 511–522. [CrossRef] [PubMed]
12. Bolcato, V.; Franzetti, C.; Fassina, G.; Basile, G.; Martinez, R.M.; Tronconi, L.P. Comparative study on informed consent regulatio in health care among Italy, France, United Kingdom, Nordic Countries, Germany, and Spain. *J. Forensic Leg. Med.* **2024**, *10* 102674. [CrossRef] [PubMed]
13. Sebastian, A.; Wyld, L.; Morgan, J.L. Examining the variation in consent in general surgery. *Ann. R. Coll. Surg. Engl.* **2024**, *106* 140–149. [CrossRef] [PubMed]
14. Jha, A.K.; Prasopa-Plaizier, N.; Larizgoitia, I.; Bates, D.W. Patient safety research: An overview of the global evidence. *Qual. Sa Health Care* **2010**, *19*, 42–47. [CrossRef] [PubMed]

healthcare

MDPI

Viewpoint

Reconciling Safety and Safeguarding in Health and Social Care: Implications for Just Culture

Siobhán E. McCarthy

Graduate School of Healthcare Management, RCSI University of Medicine and Health Sciences,
D02 YN77 Dublin, Ireland; smccarthy@rcsi.ie

Abstract: Facilitating a just response to staff involved in patient safety events is complex, with varying perceptions of safe behaviour and practice across settings. This viewpoint paper explores the challenges of developing a just culture, particularly in safeguarding situations involving peer-to-peer harm. It argues that established just culture principles, such as balancing staff and organisational accountability and using After Action Review (AAR) debriefs, need to be tailored to these contexts. In particular, organisational accountability is paramount in safeguarding situations, especially where individuals do not have the capacity to understand or intend their behaviours. Furthermore, AARs are inappropriate incident responses for serious aggression, violence, and abuse cases. To counter this, a consistent AAR practice can be valuable for preventative learning when applied to the service user care journey and comprehensive incident learning responses. The incorporation of social workers, service users, and families can help promote learning and the prevention of events. Finally, this paper emphasises the need for consistency in core safety principles across settings and the need to tailor just cultural principles to particular contexts. Future research on the role of AAR in diverse settings is recommended.

Keywords: just culture; safety; safeguarding

1. Introduction

Just culture, discerning what is acceptable behaviour and an appropriate response, is a challenging goal for health and social care systems [1]. In theory, when an unintended patient safety event occurs, a just culture ensures that staff are not punished for actions commensurate with their experience and training but also ensures gross negligence and destructive acts are not tolerated [2]. Requirements for a just culture include speaking up, support for staff involved in events, an intolerance of unacceptable behaviour, a systems viewpoint on how errors happen, and human-centred healthcare design [3]. The concept of just culture is attractive to healthcare professionals involved in patient safety events, as it shifts the focus away from individual blame for system errors towards learning and accountability. In theory, a just culture provides a balance between individual and organisational accountability and provides opportunities for open and inclusive conversations when incidents occur [4]. Implementation requires just culture education, as well as leadership support and a plan for sustainability [5]. However, barriers to just culture are numerous [6]. Different professional groups and organisational contexts may disagree on acceptable behaviour and appropriate responses [6–8]. Additionally, hindsight bias skews judgment depending on the severity of the event's outcome [7]. Across settings, the severity of the event outcome may become known across dramatically different time frames. For example, minutes in acute settings or years in residential or community care. Using the Irish health and social care system as an example, this paper discusses how safety and safeguarding are defined across the acute, residential, and community sectors in Ireland, as well as the feasibility of realising a just culture within these settings. Finally, the potential of After-Action Review (AAR), a debriefing tool, to help healthcare teams develop a just culture and come to a shared understanding of acceptable behaviour and appropriate response is discussed.

2. Safety and Safeguarding in the Irish Health and Social Care System

In healthcare, safety is often defined as freedom from accidental injury or harm associated with healthcare [9]. Common adverse events, such as healthcare-associated infections, falls, pressure ulcers, and surgical site infections, are perceived to arise not from a patient's medical condition but from their healthcare management [10]. Common preventable adverse outcomes include increased hospital stay, disability and death, as well as psychological harm to families and caregivers and second-victim impact on staff [9]. Second-victim impact comprises the psychological, physical and professional trauma experienced by staff who are unintentionally involved in a patient safety event [11].

Despite efforts to the contrary, adverse patient safety events are increasing worldwide [9]. In Ireland, two national patient chart reviews indicated that approximately one in eight admissions to acute hospitals were associated with an adverse event with little improvement between 2009 and 2015 [12,13]. Factors affecting the growing incidence include the complexity of healthcare, ageing populations, and the continuing expansion of items considered a patient safety event [10]. In recent years, there has been a shift in focus from researching the prevalence of patient safety events to examining how well institutions and teams learn, engage in quality improvement, and manage their capacity [14–16]. For example, international patient safety research frameworks emphasise the need for real-time safety monitoring alongside the measurement of locally implementable and sustainable solutions [17–20]. This shift resonates with just cultural themes, i.e., with learning and improvement being a form of accountability for the majority of errors that arise from system factors [4]. Evidently, more disciplinary forms of response are required in the case of wilful violations.

More broadly, in health and social care in Ireland, there is a parallel shift towards designing adult safeguarding strategies that integrate with overall service user safety policies [21,22]. How these shifts resonate with realising a just culture is, as yet, unclear, particularly in situations of peer-to-peer abuse [23]. First, safeguarding is the term used to ensure that individuals in health and social care settings can live free from abuse [24]. Safeguarding is essential to high-quality health and social care [25]. It involves putting in place measures "to reduce the risk of harm, promote and protect people's human rights and their health and wellbeing, and empower people to protect themselves" [25]. People with frailty due to age, a physical or intellectual disability, an acquired brain injury, a mental health condition or persons living under coercive control are considered most at risk of abuse [25]. Examples of common types of abuse include emotional, financial, physical, sexual, and organisational abuse (i.e., systematic poor care) as well as neglect [26]. In its 2023 annual report, the National Safeguarding Office (NSO) identified 22,082 alleged abuse types within 18,290 reported concerns [27]. Psychological and physical abuse were the most common types of abuse reported. For residents aged 65 years and over, 37% of concerns related to immediate family members, 33% to peers, and 20% to staff members [27]. Potentially, as an indication of the lack of assurance around the implementation of a just culture, the report recommended the need to further explore "resident-to-resident aggression" to better understand the contributory factors and protective responses required [27]. The report stated that peer-to-peer abuse may not always be perceived as a safeguarding concern [27]. A subsequent 2024 research report conducted by the Health Information & Quality Authority (HIQA) on behalf of Safeguarding Ireland identified the need to differentiate between peer-to-peer aggression and peer-to-peer abuse. Peer-to-peer abuse was then defined as "offensive, aggressive and intrusive verbal, physical, sexual, and material interactions between service users that in a community setting would likely be unwelcome and potentially cause physical or psychological distress or harm to the recipient/victim" but experts could not agree on when aggression progresses to abuse [23]. Criteria for conducting this assessment included whether the person acted on purpose and was able to understand their actions, the feelings of the victim, the behavioural needs of the people involved, and the settings in which the incident took place [23]. Due to this emerging differentiation, guidance is required to assess the organisational antecedents of each of these behaviours, especially in contexts where people lack the capacity to understand or intend their behaviours. Future awaited policy aligned with these terms will better assist the safeguarding of residents and provide the opportunity to apply a just response. The current ambiguity risks the safety of those who do not have the capacity to choose where they live despite exposure to repeated peer aggression or abuse, or lack of behavioural support.

Clearly, challenging or abusive behaviour in health and social care may not always be perceived in a vigilant manner. There may be tendencies to medicalise, accept, or ignore these forms of behaviour and avoid organisational responsibility. For example, a recent 2025 HIQA review found that an intellectual disability service with centres across Ireland had restrictive practices, poor management of safeguarding incidents, inadequate staffing arrangements, and poor behavioural support for residents [28]. Some of the residents reported feeling unsafe in their homes due to the ongoing aggressive behaviour of other residents. Furthermore, while complaints were made, concerns remained unresolved [28]. Evidently, not knowing or initiating the appropriate response to behaviours, which in other settings may be perceived as criminal behaviour, is a challenge to just culture and, ultimately, to the rights of all residents to live free from abuse. Implementing a just response based on prevention, accountability, and meeting peoples' needs in real time should help ensure all are safeguarded. Variations in what is acceptable from setting to setting should not be permitted.

3. After Action Review as a Tool to Promote Just Culture

The Irish health and social care system has promoted AAR practice as a means to help teams come together to discuss patient safety and everyday events [15]. In AARs, discussion centres around four questions: what did we expect to happen, what actually happened, why was there a difference, and what have we learned [15]? Guidelines for facilitating AARs include respect, non-hierarchy, focus on learning and improvement, no blame, and representation of what was experienced [29]. These align with the characteristics of shared responsibility in a just culture, including withholding judgment, expressing diverse opinions, avoiding blame, team-reflective learning and identifying ways to improve [30]. AARs have formed part of incident management policy in the Irish healthcare system since 2018 and have been encouraged for use in acute and community settings [31]. AARs are recommended as a concise review option for minor or moderate incidents and may be used to debrief major incidents, complementary to other review approaches [32]. In AARs, there is a focus on equal and open participation and the entitlement of all to voice individual perspectives [15]. The establishment of AAR in the Irish healthcare system can be viewed as a challenge to the here-to-fore dominant approach to the treatment of safety issues outlined in Table 1. The discussion around mainstream patient safety has predominantly viewed it as a socio-technical issue, where individual behaviours, slips and lapses intersect with systems and infrastructure in a manner that can make patient safety events happen [33]. The challenge is that the socio-technical system has been dominated by a bio-medical model, often privileging medical and nursing perceptions of safety, whereas allied health and social work views have been less privileged [33]. Given the attempt to have non-hierarchy predominate the AAR conversation, AARs can be seen as an attempt to democratise discourse in patient safety, with all having an equal opportunity to influence the safety conversation, a shared mental model about safety, as well as follow-up actions.

Table 1. Comparison of the traditional and emerging focus of safety learning in health and social care.

	Traditional Focus of Safety Learning	Emerging Focus of Safety Learning
Areas of health and social care	Acute Care	Acute, primary and social care Integrated care
Safety concerns	Patient safety Individual events	Patient and staff safety Safeguarding Integration of safety and safeguarding Care journeys and pathways over time and across settings
Learning approach	Investigative and hierarchical focus Lengthy time frame Individual learning Comprehensive learning reports	Graded learning response options from investigative to facilitative non-hierarchical approaches Immediate facilitated learning in parallel to lengthy reviews Team learning in real time after the occurrence of events Learning linked to formal quality improvement processes in addition to comprehensive learning reports
Professional perspectives	Socio-technical focus with primacy of medical and nursing views	Socio-technical focus with equality of multi-disciplinary views
Patient and family perspectives	Closed to patients and families until end of process	Inclusive of patients and families along all elements of the learning pathway
Accountability style	Individual blame Little systemic change	Balance of individual and organisational accountability Quality improvement culture

It is noteworthy that when concerns are raised in residential settings, it is often social workers who are the first port of call to address issues. Yet, social workers operate under a high degree of uncertainty, requiring the need to balance safety with autonomy for human rights [34]. Social workers, like other healthcare professionals, will experience a second victim impact when care goes wrong, but how and when do errors become apparent? Are just responses simultaneously fair in the short and longer term, and what mechanisms can help social work teams uncover this? Thus, it is acknowledged that applying the principles of just culture is more straightforward in an acute medical setting than in a residential setting. This is due to the complexity of relations among service users, their range of care providers, and the large amount of time spent living in care settings. However, creating a culture of AAR practice, including reviewing the chosen responses to these issues (i.e., undertaking an AAR of the incident response), can promote a shared understanding of the fairness and effectiveness of responses over time.

Furthermore, it is clear the just culture principle of balancing individual and organisational accountability is difficult to apply to situations of peer-to-peer aggression and abuse, where capacity issues are involved. This principle needs to be tailored to fundamentally safeguard service users affected by these behaviours while also balancing the provision of behavioural support to those exhibiting these behaviours; organisational responsibility is important to manage capacity and resources to ensure all are safeguarded.

It is also clear that an AAR is not an appropriate incident response in situations of peer-to-peer abuse or violence, and comprehensive risk assessments, investigations, and interventions are needed [31]. However, proactively applying AARs to components of care journeys and pathways, rather than isolated events [35], may help foster a culture of ongoing team reflection in residential and home care settings. Real-time safety analysis using AARs can allow for a restorative approach by focusing on both the positive and challenging aspects of care [29]. The benefit of consistent AAR practice may be preventative, particularly regarding peer-to-peer aggression escalating towards abuse. For minor events, informal AARs (i.e., brief, facilitator-free reviews without documentation) have been found to be more readily implementable and accepted by staff [29].

AARs are primarily a mechanism for staff debriefing, and service user concerns are typically met through a separate process called open disclosure [32]. However, consistent AAR practice in settings could enable the potential for service users and their families to become involved in AAR conversations, where appropriate. Informally using AAR questions with service users and families can initiate their involvement and promote a restorative focus by understanding their perspectives and utilising these to co-design improvements. The inclusion of a range of persons affected, without compromising staff willingness to engage in AARs or overwhelming service users, will enhance learning and lead to more tailored improvements [36].

4. Conclusions

A just culture may be more difficult to operationalise in residential settings, particularly where safeguarding concerns are apparent from peer-to-peer harm. Implementing a just culture remains a challenge universally, and tools like AARs are needed to help democratise the conversation about what is safe and what is to be learned. Where behaviours are found to be destructive and wilfully violate safe practices, AARs are not the appropriate response mechanism, and a comprehensive review is required. Nevertheless, should these be discovered in an AAR, AAR facilitators and organisers must be able to transfer these issues to an appropriate authority. Promoting just culture is as much about preventing adverse events and safeguarding concerns as it is about responding to issues when they arise. Consistent AAR practice, particularly during the patient's journey, may help prevent and facilitate responses to safeguarding concerns, thereby promoting a just culture. Research is needed to compare and contrast the role of AAR in safety management and in the promotion of a just culture across various settings.

Funding: This research received no external funding.

Conflicts of Interest: The author declares no conflict of interest.

References

1. Dekker, S. *Just Culture: Restoring Trust and Accountability in Your Organization*; CRC Press: Boca Raton, FL, USA, 2018.

2. European Union. *Regulation (EU) No. 376/2014 of the European Parliament and of the Council of 3 April 2014 on the Reporting Analysis and Follow-Up of Occurrences in Civil Aviation OJ EU L 122/18 of 24.04.2014*; European Union: Brussels, Belgium, 2014.
3. Oates, A. The Restorative Just Culture Manifesto: A Call for Action. In *Restorative Just Culture in Practice*; Dekker, S., Oates, A., Rafferty, J., Eds.; CRC Press: Boca Raton, FL, USA, 2022; pp. 273–280.
4. Murray, J.S.; Lee, J.; Larson, S.; Range, A.; Scott, D.; Clifford, J. Requirements for implementing a 'just culture'within healthcare organisations: An integrative review. *BMJ Open Qual.* **2023**, *12*, e002237. [CrossRef] [PubMed]
5. Barkell, N.P.; Snyder, S.S. Just culture in healthcare: An integrative review. *Nurs. Forum* **2021**, *56*, 103–111. [CrossRef] [PubMed]
6. van Marum, S.; Verhoeven, D.; de Rooy, D. The barriers and enhancers to trust in a just culture in hospital settings: A systematic review. *J. Patient Saf.* **2022**, *18*, e1067–e1075. [CrossRef] [PubMed]
7. Shorrock, S. Reflections on Just Culture. *Hindsight* **2023**, *35*, 22–26.
8. von Thaden, T.; Hoppes, M.; Li, Y.; Johnson, N.; Schriver, A. The perception of just culture across disciplines in healthcare. In Proceedings of the Human Factors and Ergonomics Society Annual Meeting, San Fransisco, CA, USA, 16–20 October 2006; Volume 50, pp. 964–968.
9. World Health Organization. *Global Patient Safety Action Plan 2021-2030: Towards Eliminating Avoidable Harm in Health Care*; World Health Organization: Geneva, Switzerland, 2021.
10. Vincent, C.; Amalberti, R. Safety in healthcare is a moving target. *BMJ Qual. Saf.* **2015**, *24*, 539–540. [CrossRef] [PubMed]
11. Busch, I.M.; Moretti, F.; Purgato, M.; Barbui, C.; Wu, A.W.; Rimondini, M. Dealing with adverse events: A meta-analysis on second victims' coping strategies. *J. Patient Saf.* **2020**, *16*, e51–e60. [CrossRef] [PubMed]
12. Rafter, N.; Hickey, A.; Conroy, R.M.; Condell, S.; O'Connor, P.; Vaughan, D.; Walsh, G.; Williams, D.J. The Irish National Adverse Events Study (INAES): The frequency and nature of adverse events in Irish hospitals-a retrospective record review study. *BMJ Qual. Saf.* **2017**, *26*, 111–119. [PubMed]
13. Connolly, W.; Rafter, N.; Conroy, R.M.; Stuart, C.; Hickey, A.; Williams, D.J. The Irish National Adverse Event Study-2 (INAES-2): Longitudinal trends in adverse event rates in the Irish healthcare system. *BMJ Qual. Saf.* **2021**, *30*, 547–558. [PubMed]
14. Lachman, P.; Linkson, L.; Evans, T.; Clausen, H.; Hothi, D. Developing person-centred analysis of harm in a paediatric hospital: A quality improvement report. *BMJ Qual. Saf.* **2015**, *24*, 337–344. [PubMed]
15. McCarthy, S.E.; Hogan, C.; Jenkins, L.; Schwanberg, L.; Williams, D.J.; Mellon, L.; Walsh, A.; Keane, T.; Rafter, N. Videos of simulated after action reviews: A training resource to support social and inclusive learning from patient safety events. *BMJ Open Qual.* **2023**, *12*, e002270. [CrossRef] [PubMed]
16. Ginsburg, L.; Easterbrook, A.; Geerts, A.; Berta, W.; van Dreumel, L.; Estabrooks, C.A.; Norton, P.G.; Wagg, A. 'We listened and supported and depended on each other': A qualitative study of how leadership influences implementation of QI interventions. *BMJ Qual. Saf.* **2025**, *34*, 146–156. [PubMed]
17. Pronovost, P.J.; Goeschel, C.A.; Marsteller, J.A.; Sexton, J.B.; Pham, J.C.; Berenholtz, S.M. Framework for patient safety research and improvement. *Circulation* **2009**, *119*, 330–337. [CrossRef] [PubMed]
18. Vincent, C.; Burnett, S.; Carthey, J. *The Measurement and Monitoring of Safety: Drawing Together Academic Evidence and Practical Experience to Produce a Framework for Safety Measurement and Monitoring*; The Health Foundation: London, UK, 2013.
19. Chatburn, E.; Macrae, C.; Carthey, J.; Vincent, C. Measurement and monitoring of safety: Impact and challenges of putting a conceptual framework into practice. *BMJ Qual. Saf.* **2018**, *27*, 818–826. [CrossRef] [PubMed]
20. Canadian Patient Safety Institute. *A Guide to Patient Safety Improvement: Integrating Knowledge Translation and Quality Improvement*; Canadian Patient Safety Institute: Edmonton, AB, Canada, 2020.
21. National Quality and Patient Safety. *The Quality and Patient Safety Competency Navigator 2025, V 1.0*; Health Service Executive: Dublin, Ireland, 2025.
22. McIlroy, J. *Moving Forward: Adult Safeguarding in the Health Service Executive: A High-Level Review of the HSE Safeguarding Policy, Procedures, Structures and Options for the Future of Safeguarding Across all Settings*; HSE: Dublin, Ireland, 2024.
23. HIQA. *Report on Peer-To-Peer Abuse: Informing Definitions and Thresholds*; Safeguarding: Dublin, Ireland, 2024.
24. Phelan, A. Adult safeguarding in Ireland: A critical review of context and gaps. *J. Adult Prot.* **2023**, *25*, 117–131.
25. HIQA. *National Standards for Adult Safeguarding*; HIQA: Dublin, Ireland, 2019.
26. Safeguarding Ireland Abuse Types. Available online: https://safeguardingireland.org/safeguarding/ (accessed on 30 December 2024).
27. HSE. *HSE National Safeguarding Office Annual Report*; HSE: Dublin, Ireland, 2023.
28. HIQA. *Overview Report of Governance and Safeguarding in Designated Centres Operated by Sunbeam House Services CL*; HIQA: Dublin, Ireland, 2025.
29. Finn, M.; Walsh, A.; Rafter, N.; Hogan, C.; Keane, T.; Jenkins, L.; Mellon, L.; Schwanberg, L.; Valentelyte, G.; Williams, D.; et al. Applying the theoretical domains framework to identify enablers and barriers to after action review: An analysis of implementation in an Irish tertiary specialist hospital. *Saf. Sci.* **2024**, *175*, 106489. [CrossRef]

0. Van Baarle, E.; Hartman, L.; Rooijakkers, S.; Wallenburg, I.; Weenink, J.W.; Bal, R.; Widdershoven, G. Fostering a just culture in healthcare organizations: Experiences in practice. *BMC Health Serv. Res.* **2022**, *22*, 1035. [CrossRef] [PubMed]
1. HSE. *Incident Management Framework*; HSE: Dublin, Ireland, 2020.
2. HSE. *Using After Action Reviews: Guidance for Services*; HSE: Dublin, Ireland, 2020.
3. Rowland, P.; Kitto, S. Patient safety and professional discourses: Implications for interprofessionalism. *J. Interprof. Care* **2014**, *28*, 331–338. [CrossRef] [PubMed]
4. MacDonald, G.; MacDonald, K. Safeguarding: A case for intelligent risk management. *Br. J. Soc. Work* **2010**, *40*, 1174–1191.
5. Vincent, C.; Carthey, J.; Macrae, C.; Amalberti, R. Safety analysis over time: Seven major changes to adverse event investigation. *Implement. Sci.* **2017**, *12*, 151. [CrossRef] [PubMed]
6. Sterkman, K.; Dekker, S. How to Implement a Restorative Just Culture and Learning Reviews in a Conservative Industry. In *Restorative Just Culture in Practice*; Dekker, S., Oates, A., Rafferty, J., Eds.; CRC Press: Boca Raton, FL, USA, 2022; pp. 177–288.

healthcare

MDPI

Article

Restorative Just Culture: An Exploration of the Enabling Conditions for Successful Implementation

Leonie Boskeljon-Horst [1,*,†], Vincent Steinmetz [2,†] and Sidney Dekker [3,†]

[1] Netherlands Defence Academy. Isaac Delprat Paviljoen, Hogeschoollaan 2, 4818 BB Breda, The Netherlands
[2] Voqx—Innovative Safety, Willem van Oranjelaan 21, 1412 GJ Naarden, The Netherlands; v.steinmetz@voqx.nl
[3] Safety Science Innovation Lab, School of Humanities, Languages and Social Science, Griffith University, 170 Kessels Road, Nathan Campus, Nathan, QLD 4111, Australia; s.dekker@griffith.edu.au
* Correspondence: l.boskeljon.horst@mindef.nl
† These authors contributed equally to this work.

Abstract: Background/Objectives: Restorative responses to staff involved in incidents are becoming recognized as a rigorous and constructive alternative to retributive forms of 'just culture'. However, actually achieving restoration in mostly retributive working environments can be quite difficult. The conditions for the fair and successful application of restorative practices have not yet been established. In this article, we explore possible commonalities in the conditions for success across multiple cases and industries. Methods: In an exploratory review we analysed published and unpublished cases to discover enabling conditions. Results: We found eight enabling conditions—leadership response, leadership expectations, perspective of leadership, 'tough on content, soft on relationships', public and media attention, regulatory or judicial attention to the incident, second victim acknowledgement, and possible full-disclosure setting—whose absence or presence either hampered or fostered a restorative response. Conclusions: The enabling conditions seemed to coagulate around leadership qualities, media and judicial attention resulting in leadership apprehension or unease linked to their political room for maneuver in the wake of an incident, and the engagement of the 'second victim'. These three categories can possibly form a frame within which the application of restorative justice can have a sustainable effect. Follow-up research is needed to test this hypothesis.

Keywords: restorative just culture; enabling conditions; leadership qualities; second victim engagement

1. Introduction

Restorative justice is becoming recognized as an important component in the ongoing quest for improving patient safety and healthcare quality. A number of converging trends and developments are responsible for this. They include the growing acknowledgment of healthcare providers as second victims of clinical errors and incidents [1–3], which can lead to moral injury [4] and worse [5]; ethical innovations in our thinking about medical error and accountability [6,7]; data showing that honesty and disclosure are cheaper than denial and lawsuits [8]; and the realization that we cannot punish and threaten our way toward a safer healthcare system [9–12] but should be creating work climates of trust and openness [13–16]. Some of these insights have come on the back of highly public inquiries into the quality failings of healthcare [17].

Restorative responses to healthcare staff involved in incidents are becoming recognized as a rigorous and constructive alternative to retributive forms of 'just culture'. The latter have typically been offered to healthcare leaders in the form of algorithms for establishing putative culpability and typically result in warnings, suspensions, and similar sanctions (e.g., [18,19]). The effects of 'being just cultured' on staff and the organization can be deleterious. Documented outcomes in studies in healthcare and other fields show that retributive responses can undermine the mental health, engagement, and motivation of those involved [20,21]; violate the rights and exacerbate the suffering of 'second victims' [1–3,22–25]; impede or even harm organizational learning and performance [8,26–28]; increase defensive posturing and safety clutter [29]; worsen staff insularity and silence [30,31]; exacerbate inequalities across medical-competency hierarchies in healthcare organizations; and invite abuses of power [32]. Restorative practices, in contrast, have yielded demonstrable benefits for second-victim experiences in healthcare [33] for claims resolution, stakeholder inclusion, quality of recommendations, just outcomes, risk awareness, and organizational learning [6,34–37].

Restorative just culture doesn't ask so much about rules, violations, and proportional consequences but instead inquires after the impacts that an incident has had on people; the needs that this has created within and around them; and the obligations on stakeholders of all kinds that this produces [26]. Those involved may engage in processes and rituals for confession (disclosure), repentance (expressing remorse), and atonement (making things right), which can lead to (secular forms of) forgiveness, the redress of harm, and the repair of relationships of trust needed to continue working with or for each other [6]. The aspiration of accountability in this is forward-looking, attached to people's roles and responsibilities, and oriented toward setting each other up for success going forward [7,38].

Conditions for the 'fair' application of retributive mechanisms—the principles of natural justice—such as an independent judge, a 'jury' of peers, and ways to appeal the outcome, have long been established [25,39], if variably followed inside healthcare and other organizations [20]. But similar meta-analyses for the fair and successful application of restorative practices in healthcare organizations have lagged behind the reporting of individual implementation initiatives [36]. Recent case research shows the application of restorative just culture, which failed to generate significant or sustainable success, even though appropriate steps had been followed [40]. In this instance, a spontaneous restorative response was observed, but an actual restorative outcome was only partially attained, in part because of a predominantly retributive organizational setting. It was concluded that a perceived tension between punishment and learning, the dilemma of choosing between one's own career and applying a restorative response, and the price of vulnerability were among the factors hindering a sustainable restorative just culture [40].

A few applications of restorative practices within healthcare have been documented: for instance, the introduction of a Just Culture Guide by NHS Improvement. Although meant with good intentions, the focus in the Just Culture Guide on individual failing made it more of a retributive than a restorative measure [41]. Stretton [42] concludes that survey results as well as individual cases show that changes made to achieve a just culture are rather superficial and entail more symbolic than actual improvements. Based on an integrative review, Barkell and Stockton-Snyder [43] concluded that the empirical evidence regarding the application and benefits of just culture in healthcare is scarce.

On the other hand, Marrée [44] found that a restorative just culture increased safety, improved the relationship between patient and caregiver, and increased satisfaction with the way incidents are handled. Flores [45] evaluated two restorative just culture interventions using community-building circles. This evaluation showed that the interventions positively impacted interpersonal relationships; changed perspectives; fostered diverse, equitable and inclusive learning environments; addressed climate concerns such as bullying within the organization; and increased psychological safety.

According to Marréé [44], the literature points to five necessary, albeit general, conditions to successfully implement a restorative just culture, which are restorative just culture training, peer support networks, learning after an incident, disclosure, and inclusivity for all stakeholders. Kooijman [46] concluded that the Hippocratic oath, an institutional learning process after incidents, and building a community, i.e., strengthening the relationships between people, can be seen as facilitators for a restorative approach. Based on a systematic review, Murray et al. [47] found four (again, rather generic) themes that provide insights into the requirements for implementing a just culture in healthcare: leadership commitment, education and training, accountability, and open communication. They also conclude, however, that most published literature regarding just culture is theoretical and that more research into requirements is necessary in order to reach a sustainable restorative just culture.

After conducting a scoping review, Sawin et al. [48] found barriers that hamper the implementation of a restorative just culture, which included historical hierarchies in an organization, the required investment of time and resources into restorative justice, resistance and opposition to restorative approaches, and longstanding traditions that favor a retributive approach. Takser, Jones, and Brake [49] identified unfamiliarity with the concept of just culture, the management of incidents and incident reports, and a lack of formal training for investigators as barriers to achieving a just culture.

Wailling et al. [50] concluded, however, that although benefits of a restorative approach can be found, the same cannot be said for the identification of specific preconditions for a restorative just culture, which is required to achieve a successful implementation. Notwithstanding the few cases reported, the literature on the application of restorative just culture paradigms in healthcare is sufficiently sparse to encourage further exploration of possible commonalities in the conditions for success across multiple cases. Although a positive change in the just culture has been observed within healthcare organizations, the conditions necessary to not only start such a change but make it sustainable remain unclear [36]. In this paper, we conduct the first empirical exploration of such enabling conditions—the kinds of conditions or capacities that need to be in place, or constraints that need to be managed effectively, to form a frame within which the application of restorative justice can be successful.

2. Method

For the current paper, we used an exploratory approach combining published cases of restorative or retributive responses to incidents in healthcare as well as other fields [20,34–37,51,52]. We needed to be fairly open-minded about which fields of practice to include, given the tiny number of documented cases in healthcare alone. Given that these published cases do not explicitly talk about 'enabling conditions', and that all took place within one field or setting without the possibility of formal or systematic triangulation with other empirical material, we elected to test our initial gleanings from these published sources against our experiences with four unpublished (operational) cases. More specifically, we reviewed published cases in the literature to gain an idea, followed by a thorough review of published cases that we were involved in as researchers, and compared these to the four unpublished cases, of which we have in-depth knowledge as a result of our involvement. As part of this exploratory approach, we distilled enabling and hampering conditions regarding a restorative just culture and elicited general themes from these that seem to provide enabling conditions for successfully implementing a restorative just culture.

Our review consisted of several rounds. After getting a basic idea from the literature, the first level of analysis consisted of the open coding of the transcripts of our published and unpublished cases. Relevant findings were marked. In the second level of analysis, comparison of the relevant findings resulted in underlying themes. Finally, these themes resulted in the enabling conditions that seem to be needed for the successful implementation of a restorative just culture.

The details of the three published and four unpublished cases are as follows: the three published cases, of which we have in-depth knowledge, come from the Dutch defense organization, as do two of the four unpublished cases. One of the unpublished cases is a case from a healthcare organization (hospital) in the Netherlands, and the last of the unpublished cases comes from a European airline.

Two of the authors have been an observer or facilitator in the aftermath of the incidents described (LBH: the three published cases and unpublished cases 2 and 3; VS: unpublished case 1 and 4).

Published case 1 contains a case study based on in-depth individual and focus group interviews, as well as observations. Published case 2 contains a case study based on in-depth individual and focus group interviews, as well as observations. Published case 3 contains a case study based on in-depth individual interviews. Unpublished case 1 contains a case study in which the author was involved in the initiation of the restorative just culture process as an alternative to the initially proposed complaint process. Unpublished case 2 contains a case study based on an interview with an involved operator. Unpublished case 3 contains a case study based on a restorative meeting with the involved parties. Unpublished case 4 contains a case study detailing a process (flight replay) developed by the operator, its safety department, and the pilots' union. The author (VS) chaired numerous replays.

These seven published and unpublished cases all contained and lacked elements which, prima facie, would have constituted important enabling conditions for restorative justice to succeed. In lieu of experimental design, the make-up of the additional unpublished cases allowed us to begin to test and control for possible confounds in the reported studies.

The published cases were as follows:

Case 1: Safety standdown: A pilot made judgement calls that made his CO doubt his capabilities. The CO sat down with him to hear his side of the story. He was satisfied with the pilot's explanations, remorse, and sense of responsibility, and the pilot received no official warning. In the months following, the pilot noticed that he was the source of gossip, resulting in the CO's decision to hold a safety standdown (A safety standdown is a RNLAF intervention that cancels all flights and brings the aviation community of a squadron together to discuss the safety matters at stake). During this safety standdown, the pilot expressed remorse about betraying the trust of his colleagues and made a public promise to do all he could to keep everyone on board safe. After his story, the responses from his colleagues showed understanding, compassion, and acknowledgement [40].

Case 2: Fatigue: During tactical training missions, the entire unit slept in tents, mimicking a situation close to the front of a conflict zone, resulting in an increasingly fatigued flight crew due to sleep disturbances. Although having been addressing this problem for five years, flight crews felt they had not been taken seriously, and they had recently been threatened with personal consequences for their careers if they did not drop the matter. The flight crews had asked for fatigue management rules dictating the sleeping arrangements and both quantity and quality of sleep. Although fatigue management rules were not provided, measures were taken for some of the future training missions [53].

Case 3: WhatsApp: A few years ago, a group of military students expressed their frustration with classes, exams, grades, and teachers in a class WhatsApp group, adding humor to these situations by using pictures and photos. At one point, some military students inserted photos of themselves and teachers into World War II imagery using photoshop. The images were eventually shared outside the WhatsApp group with the defense organization as part of a standalone legal process. The military students were threatened with immediate dismissal and a thorough investigation was conducted. Although the military students were not fired, they did face disciplinary consequences [54].

The four unpublished operational cases were as follows:

Case 1: Surgical: An infant, born with multiple congenital conditions, was dependent on constant medical care and regular surgery. The infant's life expectancy was low. Complications arose after one particular surgery and were the reason for additional surgical intervention. The infant died shortly after this subsequent surgery. The parents were dissatisfied with the disclosure and explanations the hospital gave them, and they threatened to sue. The hospital then offered a conversation with a retired surgeon, who had no connection to or interest in the clinical process, and who was not involved with this hospital. This surgeon was in a position to address the parents' questions and concerns. As a result of this conversation (even though the actual medical team was not involved, which is usual for restorative processes or alternative dispute resolution), the family was able to accept the unexpected sudden death of their child as a plausible outcome of the medical care given and was able to start the process of coming to terms with the loss [55].

Case 2: Dangerous goods: A worker specialized in transporting dangerous goods by air was ordered by his supervisor to send a load that was not properly packed nor labelled. Although this non-compliance was pointed out to the supervisor six times by the worker, the load was transported anyway. When the package arrived at the destination, the relevant authority was—by sheer coincidence—conducting an inspection. The findings regarding this particular load resulted in fifteen fines for the worker, each fine worth up to EUR 1500. The fines were rescinded later, but the situation was upsetting and frightening for this worker, who had tried everything possible within their employment relationship to 'say stop' [56].

Case 3: Air traffic management: An incident occurred in which the primary voice communication system used by air traffic controllers was becoming increasingly unreliable: instances started occurring where the system would fail completely, with aircraft flying around, unable to contact the controllers. Because of the technical issues, flight traffic was reduced but not ceased—which is what the controllers had requested. They were left feeling pressured to perform their job with an ill-working system and feared an accident could occur for which they would feel (and probably be made) responsible. Although they voiced their concerns frequently and every technical issue was duly reported, they felt unheard, their opinions, experience, and expertise not taken seriously by the organization. They felt trapped in their situation; even after the technical issues were solved, the uncertainty and fear as well as resentment towards senior management persisted [57].

Case 4: Flight crew replay: Flight operations sometimes put crews before unusual situations to which they need to adapt (against the background of goal interactions, time pressures, and limited resources), and not always with adequate procedural guidance from their organization [58]. Surprises or minor operational mysteries in such cases are not uncommon [59], leaving the parties involved with unanswered questions. A major European airline developed a method to bring multiple data traces and human perspectives together by visualizing (or replaying) relevant portions of the flight and second-to-second aircraft systems status. For this to be successful, parties have understood that several preconditions need to be met to ensure full disclosure during the replay. The critical precondition is the a-priori agreement that no other safety or disciplinary investigation will be started once a crew has requested or been invited for a replay [60].

3. Findings

Our findings elicited eight enabling conditions whose absence or presence either hampered or fostered a restorative response. They seemed to coagulate around leadership qualities, media and judicial attention, engagement of the 'second victim', and leadership apprehension or unease linked to their political room for maneuver in the wake of an incident.

Table 1 shows a few examples of the first and second analysis, resulting in eight enabling conditions (themes) that were reduced to the final three enabling conditions for successful implementation of a restorative just culture. We present the eight in more detail below.

3.1. Leadership Response

Leadership has the power and ability to choose how to respond to an occurrence. With this choice, leadership has determined the message it wants to send to its employees, upper management and/or executive board, and other stakeholders. As the studied cases show, it is not always a deliberate decision to respond retributively. Often, this is the result or outcome of a number of more or less unconsciously made decisions. For instance, the shock that leaders experience following an occurrence can result in an emotional bias. As found in the WhatsApp case, leadership, horrified by the images, immediately labeled the involved students as right-wing extremists. This was, however, not the case. Leadership was shown the end result of a process that went on for months and in which the images worsened gradually. Furthermore, the content of the images was related to the specific subject presented in class, which happened to be World War II, and not to the political affiliation of the students. Not being aware of the gradual process and context in which these images were shared, leadership responded, understandably, based on their own moral conviction instead of understanding the context surrounding the behavior and judged this behavior as both immoral and right-wing extremist [54,61–63].

Table 1. The process of analysis, resulting in 8 themes and 3 enabling conditions.

Example Findings (First Round of Analysis)	**Cases**	**Themes (Second Round of Analysis)**	**Enabling Conditions (Final Round of Analysis)**
Upper management experienced severe shock as a result of the pictures. Despite the fact that the content of the WhatsApp group for the cadets was about the humorous element and dealing with boredom and frustration, from the organization, the behavior is labelled as right-wing extremist, racist, transgressive, hurtful, insulting and referring to Nazi Germany.	WhatsApp	Leadership response	Leadership qualities
Despite the amount of pressure, there was very little support from management to help resolve the situation. Rarely did they feel there was support, which made them feel very alone. Although the problem had escalated towards management, nothing was done.	Air traffic management		
Responding in a soft, restorative way poses the risk of derailing one's career. If COs want to impress their superiors by showing how they personally managed tricky situations, retribution looks better. At the same time, COs feel that when something negative happens, they can no longer be the leaders they aspire to be. Decisions on what should be done are made higher up the chain of command and the COs are tasked with executing the wishes of their superiors without having any say in the matter.	Safety standdown	Leadership expectations	
A good example of the lack of psychological safety in a retributive just culture is the tactical training exercise that in the end permitted operators to sleep in buildings instead of tents. According to the operators, this was possible because the exercise leader had no intention of pursuing a career in the RNLAF and did not care how this decision would affect his image within his chain of command	Fatigue		
The parents and family had many open questions which the medical team tried to answer them from their perspective, medical knowledge and available information. The family, however, did not accept the explanation given and desired more and foremost better answers to their questions. [. . .] The retired doctor gave the family time and opportunity to give their perspective of their child and how they perceived the medical situation from birth till death.	Surgical	Perspective of leadership	
The exact cause, context and intention of the WhatsApp photos has not yet been investigated. However, it has been decided in advance that dismissal of those involved, which are also unknown at the time, is appropriate, despite the warnings not to look solely at political and publicity interests as this does not do justice to the situation.	WhatsApp		
After five years of trying, the operators gave up on the matter, no longer spoke up about the risks they encountered because of the belittling comments and their fear.	Fatigue	'Tough on content, soft on relationships'	
I did a PowerPoint presentation with a timeline to show exactly what happened, thinking it would lead to a better understanding of my situation. But I had to face some upsetting comments, which made me feel cornered.	Safety standdown		

Table 1. *Cont.*

Example Findings (First Round of Analysis)	Cases	Themes (Second Round of Analysis)	Enabling Conditions (Final Round of Analysis)
Communication from defense in the media and towards the Lower House shows that the first focus of top management is on taking action. The interview data show that in the perception of the interviewees, the focus is on coming across decisively to politicians and the media, a clear message that the Ministry of Defense considers such behavior unacceptable and will act harshly against it.	WhatsApp	Political, public, and media attention	Fear and unease and the political room for maneuver
Deciding 'I won't do it' is a very difficult decision when there is so much pressure regarding the progress of military operations at the airports and commercial air traffic at Eindhoven. In theory, you may and can say 'stop', but in practice you hardly do so.	Air traffic management		
The situation evolved into a conflict between the family and medical team, ending with the threat of juridical measures initiated by the family.	Surgical	Regulatory or judicial attention to the incident	
The observations made by the KMGCS led to 15 citations against the person concerned and each of these citations could mean 1500 euros fine.	Dangerous goods		
See examples above	Fatigue	'Tough on content, soft on relationships'	Second-victim moral engagement
See examples above	Safety standdown		
Pilot X acknowledged his role in the occurrence and expressed his sincere remorse, both of which made him feel very uncomfortable. [. . .] And when it was time to ask questions, there were hardly any, mostly comments that showed understanding, compassion, and acknowledgement.	Safety standdown	Second-victim acknowledgement	
It was eventually decided to dismiss the case saying that this should never happen again. The person concerned literally never did another transport. He now works in another field. The person concerned never wants to have another conversation with his former manager because there was never any acknowledgement of his situation or repentance/remorse from his manager.	Dangerous goods		
A session where crews are willing to give as much disclosure as possible about their perspective of the situation. [. . .] Once the crew is invited for a Replay, no other safety or disciplinary investigation will be started any more. Even not about what is disclosed during the Replay session.	Flight crew replay	Safe possibility of full disclosure	
Operators felt that from a certain rank up, commanding officers were reluctant to allow crew to speak up about difficult matters. Metaphorically this behavior is called the watermelon syndrome: what is red on the inside—the operator level—becomes green on the outside—the level of airbase commander.	Fatigue		

3.2. Leadership Expectations

On other occasions, the decision to act retributively is deliberately taken because it seems this is the behavior expected in the organization that the leadership is part of. Specifically in hierarchical organizations, the quality of leadership is determined by competences such as decisiveness and task orientation [64]. Dealing with occurrences in a decisive manner therefore has a positive impact on one's own career. This decisive response is more often than not translated into showing all parties involved and the rest of the organization that the behavior is unacceptable and is met with consequences. This means leadership experiences a pressure to punish [40]. At the same time, a restorative response can be quite difficult as it seems to go against what is expected: a firm response showing strong leadership. Having an example of the benefits of a restorative response can counter this unease. The safety standdown case [40] shows the power of a restorative response, as trust and relationships were restored, and the involved operator often uses this example to teach others.

3.3. Perspective of Leadership

What all retributive cases reviewed have in common is that leadership often looks at an occurrence from only one perspective: their own. However, there are different perspectives regarding an occurrence. Realizing that these different perspectives exist opens up the possibility of a restorative response [65,66]. In the surgical case analyzed, the perspective of the parents was positioned next to the medical perspective provided by the retired physician based on the medical records available. What became clear was that for the parents, living with the medical situation of their child for years, surgery was just another aspect of their normal daily routine as they had gotten 'used' to the situation over time. The medical perspective, provided in plain language, showed the parents how exceptional the medical conditions of their child were and that complete recuperation was never possible. It was known that new medical complications would arise over time with the child getting older and growing. With both the family and medical perspective of the life of the child, the family started to realize that their child lived a very special and fragile life that was not expected to last long. With the gained insights of both perspectives, the family started to accept that the unexpected sudden death of the child was a realistic possibility as an outcome of the medical care given. After the conversation, the family was able to accept the tragic outcome and start with the process of grieving [55].

3.4. Tough on Content, Soft on Relationships

A number of cases reveal an unease felt when speaking up about a situation or the 'right course of action'. In an earlier published case regarding fatigue among military pilots [53], it became clear that speaking up about the effects of sleeping arrangements on flight safety had a negative impact on how the operators reporting this matter were treated. The fact that management did not agree on the substance of the fatigue issue affected the relationship it had with these employees. As a result of this deteriorating relationship, these employees became more and more reluctant to come forward with safety-related information. They felt they were punished for their outcry. The same effect was found in the safety standdown case [40], in which an operator publicly spoke about an occurrence he had been involved in and was subsequently met with disapproval and disdain from his colleagues.

3.5. Political, Public, and Media Attention

Another finding distilled from the cases analyzed pertains to the fear and unease experienced after an occurrence, especially by leaders and upper management. If an occurrence goes public and a (negative) response from politicians and/or the media is to be expected, decisions on how to deal with the occurrence seem to be driven by that prospect [67,68]. Leadership is often pretty good at predicting a possible negative response from the public, press, and/or politicians. For instance, the analysis of the WhatsApp case shows a fear of political backlash if the case was not handled decisively, visible in the statement made public by the Ministry of Defense, in which the measures to be taken against the students and a member of leadership were announced [54]. However, in the newspapers, a news item appeared entitled, "How investigation into Nazi statements within the army was sabotaged," reporting that the defense organization is worried about its appeal to right-wing radicals and including the quote, "Those statements back then were really racist, there's no doubt about that." This media attention led to questions in Parliament.

3.6. Regulatory or Judicial Attention to the Incident

In many instances, an incident is accompanied by the (fear of the) possibility of a regulatory or judicial response, be it from outside an organization, i.e., public prosecution, or inside an organization or sector, i.e., being disciplined internally or facing professional disciplinary law. The fear of being prosecuted or disciplined results in less openness about an incident [14,69–71] and naturally hampers the possibility of restorative justice. The possibility of public prosecution is something that in most cases falls outside the scope of influence of an organization. However, judicial attention to an incident within an organization is not. The organization itself can still choose how to respond. As the surgical case [55] shows, understanding and openness to the questions and concerns of those impacted by the incident enabled eventual restoration: the family initially rejected explanations provided by the hospital, and their desire for more and foremost better answers to their questions created a conflict between the family and the medical team, resulting in the threat of suing. Instead of countering this threat by following formal complaint procedures or consulting the hospital lawyers, the hospital responded by offering an explanation via a third, unbiased party, regardless of the time (and therefore costs) needed. The tension between the family and the hospital was alleviated, and restoration became possible.

3.7. Second-Victim Acknowledgement

An important aspect of the restorative response is being aware of the suffering and needs of the people directly involved in the occurrence. These people are called second victims: practitioners involved in an incident that has an impact on someone else and for which they feel personally responsible [22]. As the safety standdown case shows, involving these second victims is key if recovery, learning, and restoring trust are the goals to be achieved [40]. During this safety standdown, the second victim, up to that point harshly judged by his peers, was provided the opportunity to share his perspective on the occurrence. Although originally intended for the second victim to provide information about the reasons behind his behavior that led to the occurrence, he took this opportunity to express remorse, making an honest apology to his colleagues for betraying their trust and accepting accountability for the situation. Although it was not specifically asked for, the second victim was forgiven and trust among the entire group of peers was restored [40]. The acknowledgement of the second victim resulted in this unit being able to compare perspectives, learn from what happened, and come to an understanding regarding future operations. Quite the opposite happened in the dangerous goods case, where the second victim was not acknowledged. In this case, the worker was not given the opportunity to share his side of the story when working with the load to be transported or the impact of the initial punishment (15 fines). The resulting fear and feelings of betrayal led to the worker experiencing a burn out, needing psychiatric help, and leaving his profession. In 2023, he left the organization, mourning the loss of team spirit he was so proud of before the dangerous goods case happened [56].

3.8. Safe Possibility of Full Disclosure

Those who are involved in an undesired event have valuable knowledge about what happened. For others and organizations to understand the course of the event, it is important that those involved are willing to disclose their narrative. Disclosure from the perspective of a restorative just culture is the ethical obligation of those involved with an adverse event to give account of that event, based on a fiduciary relationship: "Disclosure can be seen as a marker of professionalism" [26]. Disclosing one's perspective openly, after a breach in trust, is not a given. The uncertainty of what consequences a disclosure might have for the involved can hamper full disclosure [26]. To reduce the uncertainty and manage expectations, a reference framework is a necessity.

The flight crew replay case shows that an organization must acknowledge the expertise and experience of its employees as well as show a desire to attain full disclosure. The perspectives of professionals are gathered and used to make sense of (quantitative) data and events. Notwithstanding the preconditions met to ensure full disclosure, the message sent to employees that their insights are valued becomes a precondition in itself. Being seen as a professional with valuable knowledge and contributions creates a climate in which these same professionals are willing to share information and diminishes the chance that the message is met with a retributive response.

Receiving acknowledgement as a professional alone, however, was insufficient for a full disclosure. For flight replays, these aspects helped enable open disclosure:

- A written and mutually acknowledged agreement between the employer and those involved (or representatives, e.g., a union) about the replay process and its rules.
- The session is organized and hosted by a representative of an independent department within the organization: for example, the Safety Department.
- Participants are the crew, the host, a representative of the operator, and a referee, who monitors the replay being executed according to the written process.
- The crew involved with the event can ask others (except the host, who is almost always a crew member too) to leave the room if they want to disclose sensitive information.
- Information that is disclosed during the session will not be used in any written report, nor will it be traceable to the specific crew.
- When a crew participates in a replay session, it will be impossible to start any disciplinary process against the crew afterwards, nor a safety investigation [60].

4. Discussion

The analysis of the published and unpublished cases elicited eight aspects that provide insights as to what preconditions are needed to achieve restorative success. These eight aspects are: (1) leadership response, often determined by a number of more or less unconsciously made decisions based on, for instance, the shock that leaders experience following an occurrence; (2) leadership expectations, involving the decisiveness and task orientation expected of leadership in the organization, often resulting in a pressure to punish; (3) perspective of leadership, often the only perspective taken into account, ignoring the other perspectives involved; (4) 'tough on content, soft on relationships', in which speaking up about something results in deteriorating relationships; (5) public and media attention, which is the fear and unease about (the possibility of) an occurrence going public and attracting unwanted attention from politicians, the public, and the media; (6) regulatory or judicial attention to the incident, which is the (fear of the) possibility of a regulatory or judicial response from in and/or outside an organization, like disciplinary law or public prosecution; (7) second-victim acknowledgement, which involves being aware of the suffering and needs of the people involved in an occurrence that has an impact on someone else and for which they feel personally responsible; and (8) possible full-disclosure setting, focusing on freely sharing relevant information as well as accountability of all involved. Based on these aspects, we provide an in-depth discussion of preconditions for restorative success in this chapter.

4.1. Leadership Qualities

Considering aspects such as leadership response, leadership expectations, the perspective of leadership, and the 'tough on content, soft on relationships' attitude, it becomes clear that responding to an incident can be quite a challenge for leadership. The pressures on leadership to act visibly and decisively following an incident can be considerable. For instance, there is the immediate demand for damage control, for mitigation, and for preventing even worse harm from occurring. An event with a bad outcome is likely an economic issue. There can be immediate consequences of a disruption or delay in operations. If the incident is bad enough, work grinds to a halt on that ward or in that operating theater. The loss of an asset or personnel can occur. A regulator could even step in and stop operations, or the incident could attract the attention of other unwelcome sources. This means the event can be a reputational issue too, and even one of job security for the leadership.

This makes it attractive to single out and blame the individual(s) involved, focusing on what they have allegedly done wrong and what they deserve [22]. Leaders can even be seduced by the notion that acting in such a way can be sold in the name of 'safety' by fixing or removing 'bad apples' from the organization [72]. If they eschew retributive decisiveness, leaders might opt for generic but superficial expressions of compassion ("our thoughts are with..."), hedging about causes ("we will fully investigate..."), or stalling on responsibility ("we will fully cooperate..."). A full treatment is outside the scope of this paper, but it is safe to say that constructive alternatives to the 'bad apple theory' have long been in circulation in healthcare, at least in theory [8,73–76], and occasionally in scripts and guidelines [77].

What do the practical attempts to implement restorative justice show? Beyond leadership knowledge of the restorative alternative to blame and retribution, a critical enabling condition is mustering the courage to act restoratively, i.e., moral courage [40]. Courage comes from vulnerability, of course: in this case, leadership vulnerability to derision, impatience, stakeholder expectations, and even active opposition. To initiate and sustain a restorative pathway, leaders need the integrity to remain committed to upholding their values and principles and act consistently and authentically with them. Of course, when confronted with obstacles and setbacks, leaders require persistence and perseverance to continue working towards their goals, as well as the ability to inspire and mobilize others for their cause—through words, actions, and personal sacrifices and examples [66,78,79].

It also requires a foundational empathy and compassion on part of the leadership: a willingness to see and feel the perspective of the second victim and to possess a genuine concern for justice and human dignity. Humanizing the people involved in the incident is necessary to recognize their impacts and needs and to begin to understand the obligations this puts on leadership. Humanizing the people involved in the incident hinges on actually getting to know the persons—the humans—behind the role or stereotype [80,81], which takes time and effort. It may also create leadership discomfort because of the realization that whereas the care may have flowed through the hands of the people who are now second victims, the harm inflicted was produced systemically, by the organization they as leaders are responsible for [75]. The people involved in the incident did not make bad choices; they had bad choices.

4.2. Fear and Unease and the Political Room for Maneuver

A restorative process can initially be met with apprehension and unease. A retributive response is a clear and decisive response, after all, which shows that decision makers 'take safety seriously.' A restorative response takes time and might lack any form of classical punishment, thus being seen by some as not morally serious. With politicians, the public, and the media watching, this can feel rather uncomfortable. An organization, especially a public sector one, can be or at least feel to be rather dependent on the image both politicians and the media have of this organization [36,82]. Management of public sector organizations need solid public relations because they need to ensure access to resources and mandates. Management of private sector organizations, on the other hand, need solid public relations to ensure customers and growth potential. The fear of a negative image as a result of an incident can be compounded by management's perception of personal vulnerability [83]. A restorative process that requires full disclosure in order to restore trust, ensure learning, and move forwards could shed unwelcome light on the role of management in the incident. A restorative process, while repairing the harm done in an incident, might cause additional damage (a deteriorated image of management) for which, management fears, there is no simple solution. An image of being unreliable or unprofessional might be unrepairable and have severe consequences, as can be seen in the resignation of a Dutch Minister of Defence and Chief of Staff in the wake of a severe accident [84,85]. Avoiding the apprehension and unease of unwanted attention from politicians and the public—a bad review, so to speak—becomes an interest of its own [86].

Dealing with these kinds of apprehension and unease is rather complex and may be solvable only up to a certain point. However, the data suggest some things that can be done to heighten the chance of restorative success. The first is to realize that in some instances the restorative process results in a situation that requires another restorative process. If, as the result of full disclosure, a relationship between people deteriorates—for instance, because one party learns about something the other party has done and considers this below the professional standard—then that aspect also requires a restorative process. Ideally, this continues until all the damage, primary and secondary, has been addressed and resolved.

When it comes to fear of reputational damage, research shows that in some instances the possible consequences of an incident are overestimated and this fear is actually unjustified [86]. One way to deal with this fear is by simultaneously testing the likelihood of and responding to possible negative consequences, which can be achieved using a tool created for crisis communication called the Wet van Pleuris (Law of Misery) [87]. According to this law, it is possible to determine how an incident will be perceived by the public and media and what is needed to effectively deal with this perception. Three variables determine how much turmoil might occur: culpability, relevance, and mediagenicity. For each variable, this tool provides several questions to determine the extent to which it exists. These questions can also be used to create a strong narrative when communicating about the incident.

The same can be said of the apprehension or actual possibility of a regulatory or judicial response, such as the application of disciplinary law or the launching of a public prosecution [88]. In the latter case, an organization has no influence on the outcome, but it can control and decide on what response to take to the incident internally, which doesn't have to be retributive—independent of what happens in the world around. Even if public prosecution becomes a reality, an organization can still respond restoratively. This means that two different processes—one retributive, one restorative—can unfurl roughly simultaneously, where the latter almost invariably helps practitioners (second victims) cope with the stresses and uncertainties of the former [22].

4.3. Second-Victim Moral Engagement

The aspects 'tough on content, soft on relationships' attitude, second-victim acknowledgement, and a possible full-disclosure setting show that the relationship between the organization/leadership and the employees directly involved in the occurrence of the incident is a critical one.

One of the failure modes of restorative justice is unwillingness on part of the 'offender' (a poor choice of words, for sure) or 'second victim' to participate in the process [89]. Restorative justice, after all, is relational and aims to repair harm and restore relationships of trust. This is, almost per definition, impossible when key stakeholders are not part of the process. Of course, second victims can have good reasons not to want to participate, and these often go back to a lack of trust in either the process itself or the people who run it or are involved in it [90]. These issues themselves then must become objects for restorative responses, but that obviously requires more work and time, as well as faith in the eventual outcome [2]. Restorative justice is necessarily inclusive and collaborative.

Moral engagement of the second victim is an important enabling condition, and not just to ensure their meaningful involvement in the process. It involves a couple of things (see [91]). First, the second victim must be helped in accepting appropriate responsibility for what has happened. This doesn't mean that a practitioner should shoulder the blame—quite the opposite. In many cases, accepting appropriate responsibility means that many others in the organization need to engage with their roles and responsibilities. They and their decisions (about equipment, procurement, deadlines, production pressures) may well have helped set the practitioner up for failure. Moral engagement is about embracing the consequences of decisions made in those roles across the organization and finding a balance of who contributed what in steering things toward a bad outcome. It also involves recognizing and acknowledging the seriousness of the harmful effects on others. It is possible to work in an organization, even for a lifetime, and not understand the effects that incidents and their consequences have for those who were affected by them [36,51]. Restoration ideally avoids such dissociation by bringing relevant people together to discuss the impact the incident has had on them and others, achieving full disclosure, and by finding ways to address the harms that came from it together.

5. Conclusions

Although a lot has been written about the theory of restorative justice or a restorative just culture, actually achieving restoration in mostly retributive working environments can be quite difficult. Conditions for the 'fair' application of retributive mechanisms have long been established, which cannot be said of the conditions for the fair and successful application of restorative practices. In this article, we have explored possible commonalities in the conditions for success across multiple cases and industries. These commonalities can be considered enabling conditions or constraints and can form a frame within which the application of restorative justice can have a sustainable effect. We found eight enabling conditions—leadership response, leadership expectations, perspective of leadership, 'tough on content, soft on relationships', public and media attention, regulatory or judicial attention to the incident, second-victim acknowledgement and possible full-disclosure setting—whose absence or presence either hampered or fostered a restorative response. They seemed to coagulate around leadership qualities; media and judicial attention, resulting in leadership apprehension or unease linked to their political room for maneuver in the wake of an incident; and the engagement of the 'second victim'.

What is needed next is a systematic review of a larger number of existing cases to see if these three enabling conditions—leadership qualities, fear and unease about the political room for maneuver, and second-victim moral engagement—can be found consistently. Furthermore, future research could focus on experimenting with these three enabling conditions in practice in order to achieve a restorative response that is sustainable. In future research, we will therefore explore, and possibly test, if these enabling conditions can be deliberately used to ensure sustainable restorative success.

Author Contributions: Conceptualization, L.B.-H., V.S. and S.D.; methodology, L.B.-H., V.S. and S.D.; validation, L.B.-H., V.S. and S.D.; formal analysis, L.B.-H., V.S. and S.D.; investigation, L.B.-H. and V.S.; resources, L.B.-H., V.S. and S.D.; data curation, L.B.-H. and V.S.; writing—original draft preparation, L.B.-H., V.S. and S.D.; writing—review and editing, L.B.-H., V.S. and S.D.; supervision, S.D.; project administration, L.B.-H., V.S. and S.D.; visualization, L.B.-H., V.S. and S.D. All authors have read and agreed to the published version of the manuscript.

Funding: This research received no external funding.

Institutional Review Board Statement: The research is retrospective, using existing data, and is non-interventional. Ethical approval for the study was therefore not required in accordance with local/national legislation.

Informed Consent Statement: Informed consent was obtained from all subjects involved in the study. Written informed consent for publication has been waived due to the fact that participant information could not be identified.

Data Availability Statement: To access the full data, a formal request can be made to the Department of Defence of the Netherlands.

Conflicts of Interest: Author Vincent Steinmetz was employed by the company Voqx—Innovative Safety. The remaining authors declare that the research was conducted in the absence of any commercial or financial relationships that could be construed as a potential conflict of interest.

References

1. Wu, A.W. Medical error: The second victim. *Br. Med. J.* **2000**, *320*, 726–728. [CrossRef] [PubMed]
2. Denham, C.R. TRUST: The 5 rights of the second victim. *J. Patient Saf.* **2007**, *3*, 107–119. [CrossRef]
3. Edrees, H.H.; Paine, L.A.; Feroli, E.R.; Wu, A.W. Health care workers as second victims of medical errors. *Pol. Arch. Med. Wewn.* **2011**, *121*, 101–108. [CrossRef] [PubMed]
4. Shay, J. Moral injury. *Psychoanal. Psychol.* **2014**, *31*, 182–191. [CrossRef]

5. Davidson, J.; Mendis, J.; Stuck, A.R.; DeMichele, G.; Zisook, S. Nurse suicide: Breaking the silence. *Natl. Acad. Med. Perspect.* **2018**, *1*, 1–12. [CrossRef]
6. Berlinger, N. *After Harm: Medical Error and the Ethics of Forgiveness*; John Hopkins University Press: Baltimore, MD, USA, 2005.
7. Sharpe, V.A. *Accountability: Patient Safety and Policy Reform*; Georgetown University Press: Washington, DC, USA, 2004.
8. Morreim, E.H. Medical errors: Pinning the blame versus blaming the system. In *Accountability: Patient Safety and Policy Reform*; Sharpe, V.A., Ed.; Georgetown University Press: Washington, DC, USA, 2004; pp. 213–232.
9. Jung, O.S.; Kundu, P.; Edmondson, A.C.; Hegde, J.; Agazaryan, N.; Steinberg, M.; Raldow, A. Resilience vs. Vulnerability: Psychological Safety and Reporting of Near Misses with Varying Proximity to Harm in Radiation Oncology. *Jt. Comm. J. Qual. Patient Saf.* **2021**, *47*, 15–22. [CrossRef]
10. Reis-Dennis, S. What "Just Culture" doesn't understand about just punishment. *J. Med. Ethics* **2018**, *44*, 739–742. [CrossRef]
11. Mason, R. *Doctors, Nurses and Managers to Face Five Years in Jail If They Neglect Patients*; The Guardian: London, UK, 2013.
12. Moran, D. I was treated like a criminal after a harmless drug error. *Nurs. Standard* **2008**, *22*, 33–34. [CrossRef]
13. Berwick, D.M. Improvement, trust, and the healthcare workforce. *Qual. Saf. Health CareSafety Health Care* **2003**, *12*, 448–452. [CrossRef]
14. Edmondson, A.C. *The Fearless Organization: Creating Psychological Safety in the Workplace for Learning, Innovation, and Growth*; John Wiley & Sons: Hoboken, NJ, USA, 2018.
15. Grailey, K.E.; Murray, E.; Reader, T.; Brett, S.J. The presence and potential impact of psychological safety in the healthcare setting: An evidence synthesis. *BMC Health Serv. Res.* **2021**, *21*, 1–15. [CrossRef]
16. Toffolutti, V.; Stuckler, D. A culture of openness is associated with lower mortality rates among 137 english national health service acute trusts. *Health Aff.* **2019**, *38*, 844–850. [CrossRef] [PubMed]
17. Francis, R. *Report of the Mid Staffordshire NHS Foundation Trust Public Inquiry*; HMSO: London, UK, 2013.
18. GAIN. A Roadmap to a Just Culture: Enhancing the Safety Environment. 2004. Available online: https://skybrary.aero/ (accessed on 1 April 2024).
19. Marx, D. *Patient Safety and the "Just Culture": A Primer for Health Care Executives*; Trustees of Columbia University in the City of New York, Columbia University: New York, NY, USA, 2001.
20. Heraghty, D.; Rae, A.J.; Dekker, S.W.A. Managing accidents using retributive justice mechanisms: When the just culture policy gets done to you. *Saf. Sci.* **2020**, *126*, 104677. [CrossRef]
21. Morgan, D.G.; Crossley, M.F.; Stewart, N.J.; D'Arcy, C.; Forbes, D.A.; Normand, S.A.; Cammer, A.L. Taking the Hit: Focusing on Caregiver "Error" Masks Organizational-Level Risk Factors for Nursing Aide Assault. *Qual. Health Res.* **2008**, *18*, 334–346. [CrossRef]
22. Dekker, S.W.A. *Second Victim: Error, Guilt, Trauma and Resilience*; CRC Press Taylor & Francis Group: Boca Raton, FL, USA, 2013.
23. Jones, J.H.; Treiber, L.A. When nurses become the second victim. *Nurs. Forum* **2012**, *47*, 286–291. [CrossRef]
24. Scott, S.D.; Hirschinger, L.E.; Cox, K.R.; McCoig, M.; Brandt, J.; Hall, L.W. The natural history of recovery for the healthcare provider "second victim" after adverse patient events. *Qual. Saf. Health Care* **2009**, *18*, 325–330. [CrossRef]
25. Seys, D.; Wu, A.W.; Van Gerven, E.; Vleugels, A.; Euwema, M.; Massimiliano, P.; Scott, S.D.; Conway, J.; Sermeus, W.; Vanhaecht, C. Health care professionals as second victims after adverse events: A systematic review. *Eval. Health Prof.* **2013**, *36*, 135–162. [CrossRef]
26. Dekker, S.W.A. *Just Culture: Restoring Trust and Accountability in Your Organization*; CRC Press Taylor & Francis Group: Boca Raton, FL, USA, 2016; ISBN 9781472475787.
27. Hugh, T.B. Back to punishment in New South Wales. *Br. Med. J.* **2004**, *329*, 1111. [CrossRef]
28. Skidmore, S.; Ferrigno, B.N.; Chen, S.; Sade, R.M. Keeping Patients Safe: Criminal Prosecution Is Not the Way. *Ann. Thorac. Surg.* **2022**, *114*, 1551–1554. [CrossRef]
29. Carayon, P.; Cassel, C.K. *Taking Action Against Clinician Burnout: A Systems Approach to Professional Well-Being*; National Academy of Sciences, Engineering, and Medicine: Cambridge, MA, USA, 2019.
30. Hugh, T.B. Laparoscopic bile duct injury: Some myths. *ANZ J. Surg.* **2002**, *72*, 164–167. [CrossRef]
31. Mizrahi, T. Managing medical mistakes: Ideology, insularity and accountability among internists-in-training. *Soc. Sci. Med.* **1984**, *19*, 135–146. [CrossRef]
32. Von Thaden, T.; Hoppes, M.; Yongjuan, L.; Johnson, N.; Schriver, A. The perception of just culture across disciplines in healthcare. In Proceedings of the Human Factors and Ergonomics Society 50th Annual Meeting, San Fransisco, CA, USA, 16–20 October 2006.
33. Case, P. Secondary Iatrogenic Harm: Claims for Psychiatric Damage Following a Death Caused by Medical Error. *Mod. Law Rev.* **2004**, *67*, 561–587. [CrossRef]
34. Allspaw, J. Blameless Postmortems and a Just Culture. Code as Craft. 2012. Available online: https://codeascraft.com/2012/05/22/blameless-postmortems/ (accessed on 1 April 2024).
35. Cohen-Charash, Y.; Spector, P.E. The role of justice in organizations: A meta-analysis. *Organ. Behav. Hum. Decis. Process.* **2001**, *86*, 278–321. [CrossRef]
36. Dekker, S.W.A.; Oates, A.; Rafferty, J. (Eds.) *Restorative Just Culture in Practice: Implementation and Evaluation*; Routledge: London, UK, 2022.

37. Turner, K.; Sveticic, J.; Grice, D.; Welch, M.; King, C.; Panther, J.; Strivens, C.; Whitfield, B.; Norman, G.; Almeida-Crasto, A.; et a Restorative just culture significantly improves stakeholder inclusion, second victim experiences and quality of recommendation in incident responses. *J. Hosp. Adm.* **2022**, *11*, 8–17. [CrossRef]
38. Berlinger, N. Avoiding cheap grace: Medical harm, patient safety and the culture(s) of forgiveness. *Hastings Cent. Rep.* **2003**, *3.* 28–36. [CrossRef]
39. Rawls, J. *A Theory of Justice*; Harvard University Press: Cambridge, MA, USA, 2003.
40. Boskeljon-Horst, L.; Snoek, A.; van Baarle, E. Learning fom the complexities of fostering a restorative just culture in practic within the Royal Netherlands Air Force. *Saf. Sci.* **2023**, *161*, 106074. [CrossRef]
41. Kirkup, B. NHS Improvement's Just Culture Guide: Good intentions failed by flawed design. *J. R. Soc. Med.* **2019**, *112*, 495–497 [CrossRef]
42. Stretton, P. The "just culture": Why it is not just, and how it could be. *Br. J. Health Care Manag.* **2020**, *26*, 304–310. [CrossRef]
43. Barkell, N.P.; Snyder, S.S. Just culture in healthcare: An integrative review. *Nurs. Forum* **2021**, *56*, 103–111. [CrossRef]
44. Marrée, C.A.J. *Restorative Just Culture and Its Contribution to Safety for Caregivers and Patients in Hospitals A Systematic Literature Review*; Maastricht University: Maastricht, The Netherlands, 2020.
45. Flores, P.L. *When "First, Do No Harm" Fails: A Restorative Justice Approach to Workgroup Harms in Healthcare*; University of San Diego: San Diego, CA, USA, 2022.
46. Kooijman, A.L. *Healing after Healthcare Harm: The Potential of A Restorative Approach*; University of British Columbia: Vancouver BC, Canada, 2021.
47. Murray, J.S.; Lee, J.; Larson, S.; Range, A.; Scott, D.; Clifford, J. Requirements for implementing a "just culture" within healthcare organisations: An integrative review. *BMJ Open Qual.* **2023**, *12*, 1–8. [CrossRef]
48. Sawin, G.; Klasson, C.L.; Kaplan, S.; Sawin, J.L.; Brown, A.; Israni, S.T.; Schonberg, J.; Gregory, A. Scoping Review of Restorative Justice in Academics and Medicine: A Powerful Tool for Justice Equity Diversity and Inclusion. *Health Equity* **2023**, *7*, 663–675. [CrossRef]
49. Tasker, A.; Jones, J.; Brake, S. How effectively has a Just Culture been adopted? A qualitative study to analyse the attitudes and behaviours of clinicians and managers to clinical incident management within an NHS Hospital Trust and identify enablers and barriers to achieving a Just Culture. *BMJ Open Qual.* **2023**, *12*, 1–7. [CrossRef]
50. Wailling, J.; Kooijman, A.; Hughes, J.; O'Hara, J.K. Humanizing harm: Using a restorative approach to heal and learn from adverse events. *Health Expect.* **2022**, *25*, 1192–1199. [CrossRef] [PubMed]
51. Jacobsen, M. Just Culture. [Youtube]. B. Jaeansch & M. Jacobsen; Ride Free Media. 2018. Available online: https://www.youtube.com/ (accessed on 1 April 2024).
52. Khatri, N.; Brown, G.D.; Hicks, L.L. From a blame culture to a just culture in health care. *Health Care Manage. Rev.* **2009**, *34*, 312–322. [CrossRef]
53. Boskeljon-Horst, L.; De Boer, R.J.; Dekker, S.W.A. Reducing gaps between paper and practice requires more than a technical alignment. *Saf. Sci.* **2024**, *170*, 106291. [CrossRef]
54. Boskeljon-Horst, L.; Snoek, A.; van Baarle, E. Straffen of leren? Just culture en het effect op leren en herstel, een tweeluik: Deel 2: Het negatieve effect van een retributieve houding op het lerend vermogen van de defensie organisatie. *Mil. Spect.* **2024**, *193*, 518–529.
55. Steinmetz, V. A surgical case. *unpublished*.
56. Boskeljon-Horst, L. In de steek gelaten door de organisatie. *RNLAF Saf. Mag.* **2023**, *4*, 33–36.
57. Boskeljon-Horst, L.; Dekker, J.J. CCCS casus; een herstelgerichte benadering. *unpublished*.
58. Fischer, U.; Orasanu, J.M.; Montvalo, M. Efficient decision strategies on the flight deck. In Proceedings of the Seventh International Symposium on Aviation Psychology, Columbus, OH, USA, 22–29 April 1993.
59. Sarter, N.B.; Woods, D.D. "How in the world did we get into that mode?" Mode error and awareness in supervisory control. *Hum. Factors* **1995**, *37*, 5–19. [CrossRef]
60. Steinmetz, V. Flight crew replay case. *unpublished*.
61. Cook, R.I. Two years before the mast: Learning how to learn about patient safety. In *Enhancing Patient Safety and Reducing Errors in Health Care: A Multidisciplinary Leadership Conference*; Annenberg Center for Health Sciences at Eisenhower: Rancho Mirage, CA, USA, 1998.
62. Long, R. The social psychology of risk, safety and leadership maturity. *AusImm Bull.* **2016**, *12*, 26–28.
63. Schein, E.H. *Organizational Culture and Leadership*, 2nd ed.; Jossey-Bass: San Fransisco, CA, USA, 1992.
64. Scott, S. *Fierce Leadership*; Little Brown: London, UK, 2009.
65. Van Baarle, E.; Hartman, L.; Rooijakkers, S.; Wallenburg, I.; Weenink, J.W.; Bal, R.; Widdershoven, G. Fostering a just culture in healthcare organizations: Experiences in practice. *BMC Health Serv. Res.* **2022**, *22*, 1–8. [CrossRef]
66. Schein, E. A new era for culture, change, and leadership. *MIT Sloan Manag. Rev.* **2019**, *60*, 52–58.
67. Elbow, S. St. Mary's Nurse Is Charged with Neglect: Medication Eror Led to Teen's Death. *The Capital Times Madison, WI*, 2006. Available online: https://www.truthaboutnursing.org/ (accessed on 1 July 2023).
68. Wade, A. Drug Death: Nurse Stood Down. *New Zealand Herald, Auckland*, 2011. Available online: https://www.nzherald.co.nz/nz/drug-death-nurse-stood-down/4O3FL3LW73SY35LNIVDDV7QIB4/ (accessed on 1 July 2023).

Kish-Gephart, J.J.; Detert, J.R.; Trevino, L.K.; Edmondson, A.C. Silenced by fear: The nature, sources, and consequences of fear at work. *Res. Organ. Behav.* **2009**, *29*, 26–28. [CrossRef]

. Costa Pacheco, D.; Isabel Damião de Serpa Arruda Moniz, A.; Nunes Caldeira, S. Silence in Organizations and Psychological Safety: A Literature Review. *Eur. Sci. J.* **2015**, *7881*, 293–308.

. Ruitenberg, B. Court case against Dutch controllers. *Controller* **2002**, *41*, 22–25.

. Alicke, M.D. Culpable control and the psychology of blame. *Psychol. Bull.* **2000**, *126*, 556–574. [CrossRef]

. Dauer, E.A. Ethical misfits: Mediation and medical malpractice litigation. In *Accountability: Patient Safety and Policy Reform*; Sharpe, V.A., Ed.; Georgetown University Press: Washington, DC, USA, 2004; pp. 185–2002.

. Lerner, J.S.; Tetlock, P.E. Accounting for the effects of accountability. *Psychol. Bull.* **1999**, *125*, 255–275. [CrossRef]

. Morath, J.M.; Turnbull, J.E. *To Do No Harm: Ensuring Patient Safety in Health Care Organizations*, 1st ed.; Jossey-Bass: Hoboken, NJ, USA, 2005.

. Wright, D.; Mackenzie, S.J.; Buchan, I.; Cairns, C.S.; Price, L.E. Critical incidents in the intensive therapy unit. *Lancet* **1991**, *338*, 676–678. [CrossRef]

. NSWHealth. Open Disclosure. 2007. Available online: https://www.safetyandquality.gov.au/ (accessed on 1 July 2023).

. Amalberti, R.; Auroy, Y.; Berwick, D.; Barach, P. Five system barriers to achieving ultrasafe healthcare. *Ann. Intern. Med.* **2005**, *142*, 756–764. [CrossRef]

). Grint, K. Problems, problems, problems: The social construction of leadership. *Hum. Relat.* **2005**, *58*, 1467–1494. [CrossRef]

). Klein, C.A.; Klein, A.B. Alternative Dispute Resolution: An Overview. *Nurse Pr.* **2007**, *32*, 15–16. [CrossRef]

1. Macaskill, A. Differentiating dispositional self-forgiveness from other-forgiveness: Associations with mental health and life satisfaction. *J. Soc. Clin. Psychol.* **2012**, *31*, 28–40. [CrossRef]

2. Weenink, J.W.; Wallenburg, I.; Hartman, L.; Van Baarle, E.; Leistikow, I.; Widdershoven, G.; Bal, R. Role of the regulator in enabling a just culture: A qualitative study in mental health and hospital care. *BMJ Open* **2022**, *12*, e061321. [CrossRef] [PubMed]

3. Lynn, L.E. The Forest Ranger: A Study in Administrative Behavior. In *The Oxford Handbook of Classics in Public Policy and Administration*; Lodge, M., Page, E.C., Balla, S.J., Eds.; Oxford University Press: Oxford, UK, 2015; pp. 1–14.

4. Keultjes, H. Minister Hennis treedt af om fataal mortierongeval Mali. *Het Parool*, 3 October 2017.

5. Waarom minister Hennis moet aftreden. *Trouw*, 3 October 2017.

6. Boskeljon-Horst, L.; De Boer, R.J.; Steinmetz, V.; Dekker, S.W.A. Aircrews, rules and the bogeyman: Mapping the benefits and fears of noncompliance. *Safety* **2023**, *9*, 15. [CrossRef]

7. Inschatten-Wet-van-Pleuris-2.0-CCA. Available online: https://crisiscommunicatieacademie.nl/wp-content/uploads/2023/02/Inschatten-Wet-van-Pleuris-2.0-CCA.pdf (accessed on 1 April 2024).

8. Michaelides-Mateou, S.; Mateou, A. *Flying in the Face of Criminalization*; Ashgate Publishing Co.: Surrey, UK, 2010.

9. Braithwaite, J. *Crime, Shame and Reintegration.*; Cambridge University Press: Cambridge, UK, 1989.

0. Ullstrom, S.; Sachs, M.A.; Hansson, J.; Ovretveit, J.; Brommels, M. Suffering in silence: A qualitative study of second victims of adverse events. *BMJ Qual. Saf.* **2013**, *23*, 325–331. [CrossRef] [PubMed]

1. Bandura, A. Mechanisms of moral disengagement. In *Origins of Terrorism*; Reich, W., Ed.; Cambridge University Press: Cambridge, UK, 1990.

MDPI AG
Grosspeteranlage 5
4052 Basel
Switzerland
Tel.: +41 61 683 77 34

Healthcare Editorial Office
E-mail: healthcare@mdpi.com
www.mdpi.com/journal/healthcare

www.ingramcontent.com/pod-product-compliance
Lightning Source LLC
Chambersburg PA
CBHW062103220926
51850CB00010B/2872
* 9 7 8 3 7 2 5 8 5 0 5 3 2 *